Beautiful Smiles, Gentle Spirits

Fetal Alcohol Spectrum Disorder A Misunderstood Problem

Margaret A. Michaud
Sacha K. Michaud

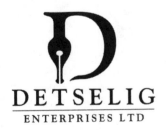

DETSELIG
ENTERPRISES LTD

Beautiful Smiles, Gentle Spirits

National Library of Canada Cataloguing in Publication Data

Michaud, Margaret

Beautiful smiles, gentle spirits: fetal alcohol spectrum disorder: a misunderstood disease/Margaret A. Michaud & Sacha K. Michaud

Includes bibliographic references and index.
ISBN 1-55059-250-5

1. Fetal alcohol syndrome. 2. Children of prenatal alcohol abuse. I. Michaud, Sacha K. II. Title.

RG629.F45M52   2003   618.3'268   C2003-910492-3

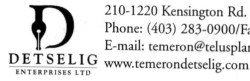

210-1220 Kensington Rd. N.W., Calgary, AB T2N 3P5
Phone: (403) 283-0900/Fax: (403) 283-6947
E-mail: temeron@telusplanet.net
www.temerondetselig.com

DETSELIG
ENTERPRISES LTD

We acknowledge the financial support of the Government of Canada through the Book Publishing Industry Development Program (BPIDP) for our publishing activities.

We also acknowledge the support of the Alberta Foundation for the Arts for our publishing program.

The Alberta Foundation for the Arts

Alberta
COMMUNITY DEVELOPMENT

COMMITTED TO THE DEVELOPMENT OF CULTURE AND THE ARTS

ISBN 1-55059-250-5
SAN 115-0324
Printed in Canada

This book is dedicated to David H. Sinclair, who taught by example that understanding, education and compassion are the necessary tools to journey successfully through life.

Acknowledgments

We would like to extend our appreciation to the many individuals, families and agencies who so generously contributed of their time and expertise to make this book possible. We would especially like to thank Jerry Marshal Adams, Robert W. Andrews, Cathy Lane Goodfellow, Pam van Vugt, Teresa Kellerman, Mary Berube and David Boulding for their contributions and the sharing of their expertise. A special thanks to Leane Maguire for her amazing multi-tasking.

A special thanks goes to Donna Anderson and Diane Wrubleski of Joining Forces, whose humor, kindness, patience and love were like a constant blanket of support as we journeyed through to make this book a reality.

We are grateful to the following people for their involvement and support: Brian R. Sinclair for his advice and graphic design input, Yuki Kurosawa for the beautiful painting on the cover, Lauren E. Sinclair for her artwork, Bruce D. Sinclair and Evelyn I. Sinclair for their continuous support and encouragement.

On a personal note, we acknowledge with heartfelt appreciation our friends and family members. Special thanks to Saleh, Ndusi, Dustyn and Chin, who so generously gave up their mother and sister to the production of this book.

Contents

Preface

We are living in a new era, the millennium, the age of instant information and the world wide web. There is ample information available regarding the recent scientific and medical findings and changes in the world of FASD.

The information that is not so readily available concerns the people who have been pioneers in this area, their struggles, dreams, hopes, hardships and successes. Birth parents, foster parents, families and friends have been care givers for FASD for years, perhaps unaware of the diagnosis of FASD, though all the behaviors were present. Pregnant women fear the negative consequences of their alcohol use and therefore often withhold accurate information. They fear being socially shamed and blamed. So many obstacles can get in the way of healthy living for the individual with FASD when we don't understand how the disorder presents itself and how to read the behaviors of secondary disabilities. Consequences can be insurmountable hurdles for the person with FASD.

In this book we will address why we see certain behaviors and how the individual with FASD views the world through different glasses. We will offer understanding and strategies for success.

This handbook offering information and understanding about FASD is not only for those who work in the community social services and criminal justice system, but also for parents, educators and caregivers. This book offers insights into a misunderstood disorder in hopes of offering improved services to those who suffer with the disability. It is intended to offer strategies and tools for an improved life for individuals with FASD, their family and community.

If you have picked up this book because you are looking for one answer or a simple solution then you should know that this isn't realistic. Through experience over several years of working in the addictions field, there is absolutely nothing simple about FASD, from diagnostic problems through to the lack of resources available. There will be a multitude of challenges in a lifetime of living with FASD.

It has been 30 years since the term FAS came to light and the only thing constant in those years has been change. Professionals in many walks, particularly medical, have been examining the issues in depth, researching safe amounts of alcohol in pregnancy and trying to come to some understanding about the degree of brain damage that occurs, in hopes that we as a society can respond more effectively.

At the onset of this project we did some random questioning regarding people's understanding of FASD. Our participants came from many walks of life, socio-economic status and educational levels. Much to our surprise, rarely did we hear same answers twice. This solidified the need for both education and understanding regarding the complicated issues of FASD. There is consensus that the disorder exists, but we lose a sense of uniform understanding in how we respond. For example, the young college student who was partying only on weekends (which relates to "binge drinking" in the FASD world) and unaware that she was pregnant at the time certainly will receive a different reaction from society than the alcoholic mom living in poverty and drinking small amounts daily. The second will probably suffer more stigma, even though the college student may have caused more fetal damage.

The truth is FASD is an equal opportunity disorder.

It does not care about care about race, age or socio-economic status.

We as a society need to destroy the barriers that prevent women from getting help – the shame and blame. We need to stop glamorizing alcohol with sports and sex appeal. We need to have available services for Canadian women with addiction concerns. What message do they get from society?

Before I (Margaret) had ever come across the term FASD, I was convinced, by what I was witnessing as an outreach street worker, that many children entrenched in the streets had unusual ways of learning and understanding. At this time I could not put my finger on the pulse of the problem due to the fact I was operating in such a difficult environment of violence, poverty, crime, and drug and alcohol consumption. It was almost impossible to know with any certainty to what the root of these behaviors could be attributed. As time went by I was convinced that there was a pattern that goes along with these behaviors, as well as repetitions of the behaviors, and that the common agent was alcohol during pregnancy.

Modern society is bombarded with science and technology, with understanding and validating human behavior through the use of tests, experiments and studies that generate statistics. We might not accept what we are seeing or trust our own experience due to the fact we have closed our minds to any approach which can not be proven or measured by the appropriate scientific tools. Questions arise, inconsistencies exist, humans differ in experience from one person to the other. You might hear people say "my sister or friend drank when she was pregnant and her child does not have FASD." In fact, this can be true but that doesn't mean that this would be the outcome for another person in similar circumstances. This is a reality when we delve into the world of FASD. As we explore we will find that there is room for individual differences due to environment, nutrition, health and circumstances. It is true that some woman may be fortunate and drink throughout her pregnancy and all is well. This does not mean it would be the case for the next person, for she may not be that fortunate.

I was delighted when I first discovered Dr. Ann Streissguth and her work in the area of FASD. The questions which she posed and her experiences mirrored my own. This purpose of this book is not to convince people of the existence of FASD, but rather to present the facts, give the information, share the stories and offer understanding.

I have been fortunate throughout my career to have encountered a number of professionals working in the area of addiction who are pioneers in the world of harm reduction and open minded to new approaches. Alcohol is the oldest drug, the one that has been used most frequently and that is legal.

Harm reduction is the newest approach and is applicable to the oldest drug.

I am thankful to share with others, to continually search for the answers and solutions, to continue to be dissatisfied with less than adequate services, to fight for the rights of those with FASD and their loved ones. Our intention is to reach out and educate for the benefit of all those children in foster homes or before the courts who live a life that is wrought with misunderstanding. It is our hope that with education and understanding comes insight and that we, as a society, can embrace better ways to assess, support and offer social programming to those who suffer with FASD and their caregivers. We must be mindful that there will always be individual differences, that the recognition of the disorder offers guidelines not set in stone and we must always be adaptable.

There is an African proverb that states "it requires a village to raise a child," and certainly this is applicable when speaking to children living with FASD. The inspiration for this book are those individuals who suffer from FASD. I am constantly moved by their beautiful smiles and their gentle spirits. During my 16 years of working with multi-barrier women and their families, many clients opened their hearts and shared honestly about how FASD has impacted their lives and the lives of their families. It was not unusual, given my line of work, to encounter a higher percentage of

FASD. It was often the case that my clients battled with poor education, poverty, drugs and other socio-economic barriers.

This book is exciting in that it brings together a spectrum of voices in the community: the professionals, medical, legal, educational and networking, with the families, caregivers and most importantly, FASD individuals themselves. This approach is intended to offer the most holistic approach to understanding and a future vision for FASD.

We hope that after going on this journey of understanding about FASD you are left with a greater optimism towards the future for all whose lives are touched by FASD. If you have a loved one who suffers from this disorder, you will find comfort in the compassionate approach presented throughout this book. This book offers support, hope and optimism from those whose lives are touched personally by FASD.

Margaret Michaud
Sacha Michaud
August 2003

Foreword

I was asked by my friend Margaret to write the foreword to her book. I have always said yes and then not written it for her. I asked myself why and I came to the conclusion that most books talk about what we have not done for youth, say that we have not listened to them, that we have not done our jobs and that we are happy to save one child out of a hundred. Why are we happy just to save one youth or child? If we were a business, we would be bankrupt by the small numbers of our successful clients.

I am doing it this time because I feel that my friend Margaret does a lot of work that is sincere, and does it in a holistic manner. Sometimes it is the simple solutions that are the most affective way of dealing with the trauma and pain of the young folks. The constant issues that come up for youth and Aboriginal youth are historical pain and issues. What does that mean for youth? They will say it is not significant, that they are hurting now so why should they listen to their parents' pain or their grandparents' pain. It is true that youth are suffering now and they also feel isolated by all that is around them. We the caregivers are doing all the right things according to what we think is right.

When I was a brand new social worker, I thought I knew everything and that I knew what was best for the child. Well, I did come to my senses one day when I thought I was listening to the youth and what her needs were. I was not listening and I was not in tune with the child's feelings either. This is how it went.

I brought a young woman to an emergency home and introduced her to the director of the home. We went through the rules with the young woman and proceeded to ask her what she wanted to do with her life. She responded by saying that she wanted to take drumming lessons, that was easy. She wanted to go to hair dressing school, even better. And she wanted to go to counseling, excellent. The director and I were beside ourselves, we could not believe how great we were and practically did cart wheels.

The young woman was probably sincere, but she had outsmarted us. She knew what we needed to be happy workers and she read us better than we understood her. She knew what our needs were and she knew what she had to do and she did it. She understood the situation and delivered what she had to do, we did not. As the other worker and I did our high fives and cartwheels, the woman walked out the front door and did not return.

What I learned was that my listening skills did not pick up what the real needs of the woman were and that she was much more astute than I was and she understood people dynamics. I feel that this is all too often what happens to our youth today. We so want to do the best for them, but at the end of the day, we have done nothing for them. The other side of our dilemma is the workers who do not care for youth at all or do not want to care about youth and choose not to understand them. I am referring to the multi-barrier youth of today. The challenges for an individual with FASD can be tenfold those of your average teenager. The teen years by nature are difficult, and coupled with learning disabilities, it is a constant uphill battle. We as caregivers need to listen to the voices of their struggles.

The book will look at why our misguided intentions are not working. I have a strong belief that youth should not be thrown into detention centres or other systems that are not supportive of youth. Having experienced it firsthand, I know it does not work. I also once had the idea that it would be a good idea to have youth incarcerated. Again it was done for them on my recommendation to ensure that they were protected from themselves and their self-destructive behavior. It seemed like a good plan at the time, but it was again not in consultation with these youth.

Why did it not work? These youth were not ready to deal with the issues that I believed needed to be dealt with.

Well-intended plans still do not work and we have to question why they are not working. The more we get specialized, the less able we are to understand youth in their plight and the more we isolate them from getting better.

This is a hard time for youth who do not have the supports that they need. They are in crisis and they are in a place of neediness. They want their families back no matter how much we want to remove them from their homes. As one young man indicated to me, he did not need to be reminded how bad his family was. The young man knew his father drank too much, he knew his father was a drug addict, but he still wanted to be with him. This situation can be further complicated when we are dealing with young people who are living with FASD. We as caregivers would be best armed to help if we had a full understanding of the complications of FASD and the impact it has upon their lives.

The issue of FASD is not new, but it is a neglected concern for children who need a place for their hopes and dreams. That can happen if given the right supports, but mainly through the love that people like

Margaret have offered for years through the work she has done with young moms and their children in Vancouver and now Calgary.

There are professionals who say this method of investing your whole heart into your work and making people trust you is not right. I say they are wrong. This trust and love is what these young people need and want.

We try to analyze the situation when, for example, they missed their appointments because they did not understand the language or maybe they just needed a bus ticket to make their appointments. We can set up barriers without even knowing that we have done it. As caregivers, we have to not guess what people want, but listen to what they are saying to us. It sounds simple enough, but it does not happen because the guiding principles are from our value system and also from our own family core beliefs.

I believe what is told in the book is not new nor is it complicated; it is tried and has worked because it is written from a place of knowledge and love. In order to work successfully with those individuals living with FASD, we must attempt to understand their point of view, combined with all the knowledge we have in 2003. Healing is a long process and it has to work for the person or persons who want to make that effort to change. Margaret has moved the boundaries by going back to dealing with the actual needs of youth and their families.

We caregivers will always be in the business of helping people and we will always need to change the way we deliver services because of the constant challenge that is presented in the face of poverty, addiction and learning disabilities like FASD. The work will forever need updates and we have to be as adaptable as they are, because at the end of it all, they are the ones with the REAL pain.

Jerry M. Adams
Executive Director
Urban Native Youth Association
Vancouver, British Columbia
August 2003

Introduction

I first met Margaret Michaud while I was working as an administrator at a Poverty Law Clinic in Calgary. We traditionally saw few sex trade workers in our evening legal clinic, and had not done much analysis around the possible barriers that had prevented them coming through our doors to access services since a targeted outreach clinic had ended a few years before. Margaret and I fell into an arrangement in which she bypassed the standard intake process and evening clinic appointments with volunteer lawyers, which seemed to either intimidate her clients or at least not meet their needs. She and I booked clients directly in to the service stream and opened files. This continued after I resigned and (finally, after a hiatus after law school) decided to complete my articles at the clinic. Margaret has brought many sex-trade workers with Communication charges, probation breaches and other legal challenges through our doors. Without her presence I am certain that many of these clients, without access to legal aid for summary conviction offences, would simply have been warehoused via guilty pleas in docket courts through the criminal justice system and criminalized as a simple matter of course.

At the time, Margaret was working (and continues to work) on the street with Calgary's sex-trade workers. What makes her practice of social work remarkable was that she literally works *on the street*. My experience has been that many "street outreach" workers spend an allotted amount of time "doing" outreach. However, Margaret's office is literally the sidewalk (and transit trains and intersections and coffee shops in the city core), usually with a client by her side on the way to or from a problem and a possible solution. That problem or solution may be a communication charge, a missed court appearance, a housing crisis, a custody crisis, a job-training opportunity, or a client in some kind of danger. That is not to say that I wouldn't be on my way to court and run into her sitting on a newspaper box shooting the breeze with a client about a great thing happening in their lives, all the while building trust and "street cred."

It is telling to note that I don't recall ever trying to call her or return a call to her in her office. I would call her cell phone and find that she was on a sidewalk on her way somewhere with a client, or a couple blocks from our office and, "well so and so that I called about is with me, and we're on our way to so and so, do you have a few minutes and can we pop over?". This is telling for several reasons. First, it reflects the level of engagement that she seems to find successful in her practice. Second, it reflects the level of detail and engagement necessary to effectively assist this group of clients and also the multiple layers of issues and challenges faced by an FASD client. No single client has a single issue such as a criminal communication charge. Every single client has a myriad of issues such as new criminal charges, probation breaches, custody and relationship complications, an imminent housing crisis and a substance abuse problem.

Ironically, in such cases the thing these issues may have in common is that they live together in a list of symptoms in this book, but are all dealt with by the criminal justice system and social services agencies in isolation. The lack of a diagnosis is one of the biggest challenges facing a person with FASD or their caregivers. It also presents an argument that the lack of diagnosis more often that not stems from the lack of a standardized screening tool, screening resources and structures for screening within the criminal justice system.

As soon as people hear about alternative sentencing theories in the criminal justice system, eyebrows are raised and the challenge emerges. However, if you have not read a great deal about FASD, expect to be challenged in other senses. It is not a surprise that poor, urban, Native women who are in receipt of social services are an easily accessed study group in the area of FASD, but it is more of a challenge to read where else in society FASD may be an explosive issue. Margaret also excerpts an excellent survival guide for parents and caregivers of FASD youth involved in the criminal justice system, by David Boulding, a Vancouver criminal defence lawyer. Many may find the conclusion of his survival strategy for parents fatalistic. It is certainly challenging, but also certainly well reasoned.

Since I graduated from law school in 1993, I have worked primarily in two marginalized environments: first, in HIV/AIDS prevention education and outreach, and then in a poverty law clinic. In 2003 as I read the draft of Margaret and Sacha's book and background material on FASD, I made the connection: patterns of high risk behavior, failing to learn from actions, inability to keep appointments and missed court appearances, failure to really grasp consequences…I have "served" FASD clients for years without the tools to properly serve their needs. My entrenched notions around the connection between systemic socio-economic disadvantage and high-risk lives are further entrenched.

Social, cultural and economic barriers to FASD diagnosis and intervention abound. Work like Margaret's must be the siren song to build on the momentum that FASD awareness needs. Momentum in this field can truly affect service for FASD individuals and families and effect broad behavioral change to eliminate fetal brain damage in utero. This work, from street level, makes the case that this momentum requires judicial education, a standardized screening procedure, resources and an accessible "port of entry" into FASD assessments within the court system, and lots and lots of perseverance. Have a good read.

Robert Andrews

Contributing Authors

Margaret Michaud is a counselor and consultant specializing in the area of harm reduction, addiction and multi-barrier women and children. Ms. Michaud has worked actively in the Downtown Eastside of Vancouver as an administrator, front line worker and group facilitator. Recent endeavors have included lecturing in several countries on Harm Reduction as an effective model to working with multi-barrier women and their children. Ms. Michaud is interested in developing innovative harm reduction programs that address the many issues related to poly-drug use, sex trade workers, HIV/AIDS and socio-economic deprivation. She is the author of *Dead End: Homeless Teenagers A Multi-Service Approach*, a book focusing on juvenile prostitution.

Sacha Michaud is a student of International Development at the University of Calgary. In 2000 she studied therapeutic massage in Maui, Hawaii. She has continued to pursue her interests of women's health and program development on both local and international levels. She is presently at the University of Pune in India. Upon her return she will be starting a theatre project working with multi-barrier youth in Calgary. She is planning on moving to New Zealand to continue her studies.

Cathy Lane Goodfellow, BA, LLB, LLM, graduated from the University of Alberta Law School in 1983 and practiced law in Edmonton from 1984 to 1991 in the areas of family law and youth criminal defence. In 1992 she relocated to Calgary and has been in continuous employment with the Youth Criminal Defence Office since October 1993. This Office practices exclusively in the area of youth criminal defence.

Cathy obtained her Master of Laws Degree in 1995. Her thesis is titled "The Philosophy of the Young Offenders Act and its Impact on the Formal Legal Education and Practice of Advocates for Youth." She has guest lectured numerous times for a variety of organizations on the topic of young offenders and the YOA. Organizations include parent support associations, High Schools, Junior High Schools, "Best Beginnings" a teen parent support agency, Victim Assistance and Native Counseling Services of Alberta. She is both a lecturer for the Legal Education Society of Alberta and a sessional instructor at the University of Calgary, Faculty of Law. Cathy shares her busy life with her husband Steve Goodfellow, step-daughters Cristy and Amanda, dog Pepper and cats Lincoln and Kohl. In her leisure time she snowboards and plays golf. Her passions include photography and being a member of the pit crew for "Goodfellow Racing." Life must have balance!

Jerry Adams has dedicated his whole career working with Youth and especially Aboriginal Youth in the Greater Vancouver area. He has been married to Linda for 29 years and they have three children. He is from the Nisga'a Nation but has spent most of his life away from his family and his Nation. He was sent to school in the Lower Mainland area of BC, because the Federal Government in the 60s had decided to start moving some Aboriginal youth away from the residential school system. He has lived in Vancouver for over 27 years and has done childcare work, family support work, outreach work and social work. Currently he runs a non-profit organization that specializes in working with street-involved Aboriginal youth in Vancouver, BC. The life of Aboriginal youth are important to Jerry and he wants to see that all children get the best possible services that can be provided to them. He is passionate about the rights of children and youth, but believes that we have not done enough to help them; as great a nation as Canada is, we are still third world when it comes to the poverty of our children and their families.

Mary Berube, BSW, RSW, is an FASD specialist in the province of Alberta. She recognized the impact of prenatal exposure to alcohol on her two adopted sons when they were ages 19 and 18 (1992), and became a passionate, outspoken advocate for families living with Fetal Alcohol Spectrum Disorder (FASD). As a social worker, Mary has translated her personal experience into training and providing family support through her program management, as well as in her role as FASD Specialist with the province. She developed and is Manager of three programs dealing with issues of FASD. Mary lends her expertise to many agencies and committees by way of reviewing new material, providing extensive training, and offering her professional support. She is called on across Canada to provide support to FASD committees in developing a response to FASD issues of practise, training and service delivery, and has presented extensively with international specialists in the areas of FASD.

David Boulding obtained an English (Honors) degree at Trent (1981) followed by a Master's degree in Modern Poetry (UBC, 1988) and then a law degree from UBC in 1988. He has been a loud participant at various environmental enquiries, including working on the Kelowna helicopter spray cases in 1989.

David has always been a trial lawyer, and yet he has always advised clients not to go to court as a first response. He has stressed principled negotiation and mediation as alternatives to appearing before a judge. He is a law society certified family mediator and has appeared in criminal courts most times as a defence counsel and sometimes as Crown counsel.

After some 13 years as a working criminal/ family lawyer, he wrote a paper in the fall of 2001 at the request of Judge C. Trueman of Vancouver Provincial Court called "Mistakes I have made with Fetal Alcohol Clients." Later, he wrote a second paper, again prompted by the same visionary judge, called "The Several Languages of Law." As a result of these papers, he has spoken at FAS conferences in Vancouver, Kelowna, Toronto and Kodiak, Alaska. He has made further presentations to various parenting groups and police forces.

David has good sense of humor, but can be "impressively obnoxious," though usually for a good cause. In his spare time, he owns and operates a small logging/milling and tree topping business. Recently he has also been helping out at the family business at Strathcona Park Lodge.

Robert Andrews is a lawyer living and working in Calgary, Alberta. After studying English Literature and Political Science at the University of Toronto, he attended law school at the University of Calgary, graduating in 1993. Throughout the 1990s he worked as both a volunteer and staff HIV/AIDS educator in schools, prisons, workplaces and on the street. He worked for a number of years as an administrator at a poverty law clinic in Calgary, and eventually completed his articles at the same clinic, providing legal services to low-income Calgarians ineligible for legal aid.

Pam van Vugt is the supervisor of the Parent Child Assistance Program (P-CAP) at McMan Community Services in Calgary. Pam worked for nine years as the Public Education Coordinator at a Sexual Assault Centre. Pam has 22 years experience as a Sexuality Educator.

Teresa Kellerman is an adoptive mother and nationally recognized parent advocate in the United States. Teresa's advocacy and tremendous sense of humor are to be applauded as she continues to be a leader in the world of FASD.

Yuki Kurosawa created the painting used on the cover of this book. She was born in Maebashi, Japan, in 1960. She moved to the United States in the 1970s, where she studied painting and linguistics. Yuki is a graduate of the School of Art Institute of Chicago. In addition to painting she also practices traditional Japanese woodblock. She lives in Calgary with her husband and five children.

Alcoholism in a Cultural Context

In most western countries drinking alcohol is a cultural norm. According to a 1995 statistic collected by the Brewers and Licensed Retailers, France had the highest per capita consumption levels at 11.9 liters of pure alcohol and Canada had the lowest at 6.1 litres (p. 15, Waterson). In the US alone, the alcohol industry caters to over 100 million citizens and yields $115 billion in annual sales. Alcohol commercials, particularly for beer, are notorious in regards to their portrayal of women. Due to the fact that children between the ages of 2 and 18 watch 100 000 beer commercials (Roth), our attitudes about women and alcohol and power are very much a part of our socialization. The media, in all of its manifestations on screens or paper, has the tremendous and unyielding ability to reflect and influence the ideals of a culture. Over the last half century, it has become an increasingly potent tool for the socialization of the young and for solidifying social norms in adults. Children are socialized to understand and perpetuate culturally exclusive attitudes about what is considered valuable in their culture. Media, along with other mediums of socialization, shape and sustain an individual's outlook on the world and the value which they place on themselves and the people they encounter. This is certainly true in relation to women and alcohol use.

As is true with many factors of human behavior, drinking has certain gendered rules. As a result, societal attitudes correlate to the sex of the drinker. Women drinking results in more consequences in all realms of life and they are targets of more blame, especially when related to issues regarding motherhood. Public attitudes related to women and alcohol are not a recent phenomenon; in ancient times drunkenness in women was punishable by death (Browne). Social controls apply to women more than men – there are more restrictions on their behavior and more judgement when they deviate from norms (p. 227, Macionis). This creates the appearance of an increased need for public supervision of women who drink, despite the fact that from a statistical standpoint men are the irresponsible sex when it comes to alcohol consumption. Women account for 5% of drunk driving offences and 7% of all drunkenness offences. Men are more likely to become drunk and involved in public disorder, criminal activities and accidents (Waterson).

Yet at the same time there is a noticeable shortage on research literature concerning the medical effects of alcohol on women's bodies. Most of the research about the health detriments caused by alcohol are based on studies in which all the research subjects were male. Between the years of 1929 and 1970, there were only 28 English language articles published about women and alcohol. Until 20 years ago, alcohol continued to be used for pain relief in labor and in preventing pre-term labor. It was also used as a remedy for infant colic – in fact, the permitted daily dose for an infant was four ounces of alchohol (Waterson).

In the last three decades, spurred by the women's movement, public demand, largely orchestrated by grassroots groups, spearheaded initiatives to increase knowledge of women's bodies, fuelling more medical research relating to women. In the last decade, more women-focused studies were conducted; despite this, Gomberg insists that women are still the "second sex" when it comes to alcohol studies (Gomberg, 1993).

Though more research has been conducted over the last 30 years, the majority of it fits into two categories; 1) drinking and pregnancy, 2) alcohol and social deprivation (Waterson). This bias, fuelled by extensive and selective media coverage, has demonized mothers who drink during pregnancy and has resulted in the perception that FASD is a disorder that is present only below the poverty line. It must be understood that this is not the case. It must be understood that persons entrenched in poverty are more visible – the research bias exists because they are more easily surveyed than the rest of the population. They are more likely to rely on social assistance, participate in social programming and require other services that increase their visibility to researchers. There is more government presence and control over their lives and the lives of their children. Just because the studies related to FASD are among women of poverty does not mean that FASD does not exist in middle and upper classes. Money and race provide the freedom to remain relatively anonymous and if problems arise, the resources can be used to escape the social scrutiny and blame. Minorities living in poverty are easy targets for social outrage and disgust.

We must challenge our collective tendency to misrepresent problems present in all groups in society, minority, majority, gender, sex, age, as being exclusive or predominantly problems associated with poverty. Not only are these attitudes not fair representations of the reality of the situation, but the blame and denial does nothing to benefit those in that situation. Our denial is detrimental to every player involved. It is unfair to categorize and victimize the poor because they are easy targets, lacking the resources or support networks to counter the claims. Denial of the problem prevents them from gaining help, because of the crippling social stigma attached to themselves and their children.

Definitions:
Understanding Terminology

In order to understand FASD, communication begins with speaking the same language; therefore we will present terminology.

What is FAS?

There has been tremendous growth in the area of FAS over the last 30 years. FAS was first described in France in the 1960s. In 1968, Dr. Paul Lemoine and his colleagues published the results of a study of 127 children born to alcoholic mothers, followed in 1973 with similar research results that appeared in the United States. These studies clearly established the relationship between alcohol abuse and birth defects. The conditions were difficult to recognize because not every woman who drinks heavily bears a child with the symptoms and abnormalities seen in FAS. At this time, advances began in our understanding of health and the disorder.

FAS was named as a birth defect in 1973 when two University of Washington dysomorphologists, Dr. K. James and Dr. David Smith, identified 11 unrelated children from three racial backgrounds with a cluster of physical and intellectual features associated with prenatal maternal alcohol consumption. The alcohol consumption during pregnancy results in damage to the central nervous system, thus causing intellectual impairments to the child. In defining FAS individuals, we are looking at three essential traits.

1. Prenatal and/or postnatal growth restriction
2. Characteristic facial features
3. Central nervous system impairment

FAS requires these three criteria as well as a positive history of prenatal maternal alcohol consumption.

Now that FAS was officially confirmed as a birth defect, further research was conducted with animals that indicated that alcohol is a teratogen which can have numerous and serious consequences on fetal development. Recent research has indicated that the glial cells, which compromise approximately half of the brain's volume and play an important role in brain development, are sensitive to alcohol and increase the vulnerability of the brain to serious damage (Lancaster).

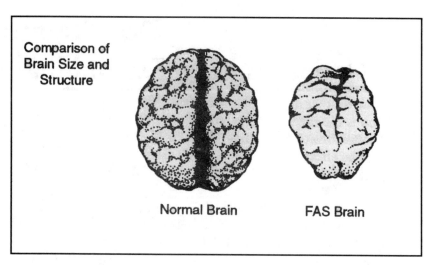

Above: A drawing comparing a normal brain, and the brain of a person with FAS/FAE. Adapted from Diane Malbin, Fetal Alcohol Syndrome, Fetal Alcohol Effects: Strategies for Professionals *(Center City, MN: Hazelden, 1993, p. 10).*

Below: Facial Characteristics of Fetal Alcohol Syndrome. From Streissguth et al., A Manual on Adolescents and Adults with Fetal Alcohol Syndrome with Special Reference to American Indians *(University of Washington, 1988, p. 7)*

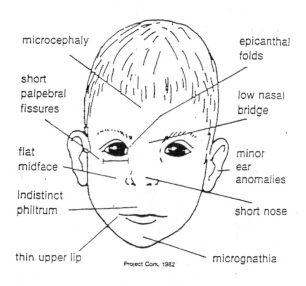

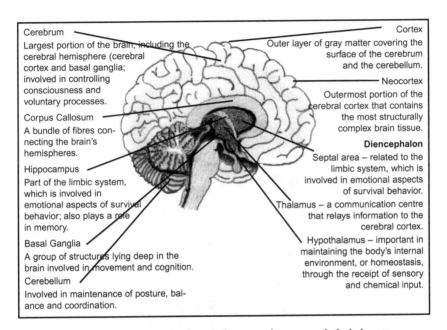

Cerebrum
Largest portion of the brain, including the cerebral hemisphere (cerebral cortex and basal ganglia; involved in controlling consciousness and voluntary processes.

Corpus Callosum
A bundle of fibres connecting the brain's hemispheres.

Hippocampus
Part of the limbic system, which is involved in emotional aspects of survival behavior; also plays a role in memory.

Basal Ganglia
A group of structures lying deep in the brain involved in movement and cognition.

Cerebellum
Involved in maintenance of posture, balance and coordination.

Cortex
Outer layer of gray matter covering the surface of the cerebrum and the cerebellum.

Neocortex
Outermost portion of the cerebral cortex that contains the most structurally complex brain tissue.

Diencephalon
Septal area – related to the limbic system, which is involved in emotional aspects of survival behavior.
Thalamus – a communication centre that relays information to the cerebral cortex.
Hypothalamus – important in maintaining the body's internal environment, or homeostasis, through the receipt of sensory and chemical input.

Areas of the brain that can be damaged in utero by maternal alcohol consumption. Adapted from Alcohol Health & Research World, Vol. 18, No. 1, 1994.

What are FAE and ARND?

Another term identified was Fetal Alcohol Effect, which was used to describe children with prenatal exposure to alcohol but who have only some of the FAS characteristics. In 1996 the Institute of Medicine published a review in which a new term for FAE was introduced, "Alcohol-Related Neurodevelopment Disorder (ARND)" (Stratton, Howe and Battaglia). The new label was helpful, for there are many individuals who are victims of this disorder, but who don't have all the facial features as indicators. Fetal Alcohol Effect is a diagnosis used when there is a known history of maternal drinking during pregnancy and when some, but not all, of the three criteria for a FAS diagnosis are present.

What is Fetal Alcohol Spectrum Disorder (FASD)?

FASD is a new term being applied to the spectrum of symptoms and disabilities associated with prenatal exposure to alcohol. In the past more weight was given to a diagnosis of FAS than FAE, despite the fact that those

The Effect of Toxic Substances* on Development

*Such as: Alcohol, tobacco smoke, illegal drug and some over the counter and prescription drugs.

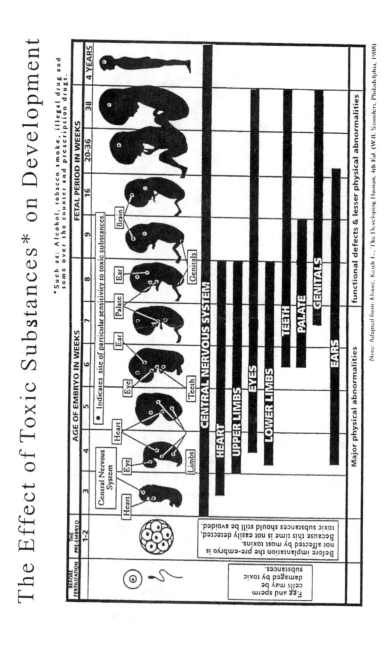

Note: Adapted from Moore, Keith L., The Developing Human, 4th Ed. (W.B. Saunders, Philadelphia, 1988)

Adapted from Moore, Keith L., The Developing Human, 4th ed. (W.B. Saunders, Philadelphia, 1988).

affected with FAE have been shown to experience more secondary disabilities related to their diagnosis. FASD, as an emergent term, will hopefully encourage the understanding that beyond the physical signs of prenatal exposure to alcohol, those affected experience serious emotional, behavioral, intellectual and cognitive difficulties.

Both FAS and FAE indicate permanent brain damage. Children with FAE are adversely affected by prenatal alcohol exposure but they do not meet the formal criteria (Matts metal,1996). As Donovan adds, these children may actually face more serious problems because their symptoms are not recognized. It was the medical term FAS that brought it to the attention of many professionals. FAS is a complex and multi-determined problem which presents a number of challenges. Abkarian asserts that FAE presents a behavioral phenotype as robust as physical characteristics in marking FAS. Through this recent research we have determined CNS damage (central nervous system), brain dysfunction and with FAS, facial dysphormology, but how does this present in terms of behaviors? Although the range of intellectual functioning varies, FAS is now considered to be the leading cause of mental retardation in North America (Streissguth et al., 1991). What is clear is that there are numerous physical, neurological and intellectual disabilities in individuals with this disorder.

Current Facts about FASD

Some additional facts are as follows: FASD is alive and thriving in the year 2003. It has been three generations since we first heard of the disorder. This is years after the government put warning labels on alcohol products, years after Health Canada saw the concerns that lay ahead, as did Corrections Canada. The fact is that alcohol is a very popular and legal drug, this society's approved drug of choice. The fact is that all women of childbearing age can be vulnerable. Having said all this, it is imperative to ask why this preventable cause of mental retardation simply doesn't disappear. In this age of information, there should be no excuse for not being informed. We believe we are informed, but the stigma our society puts on mothers of children who have been exposed to alcohol in pregnancy creates shame and blame, in turn preventing maternal reporting. Self-reporting, or lack of accurate reporting, is a weak link in diagnosis. Due to the fact that FASD still remains highly controversial, women still do not feel safe in reporting an accurate account of their drinking during pregnancy.

As a society we must change our judgmental attitudes and offer support.

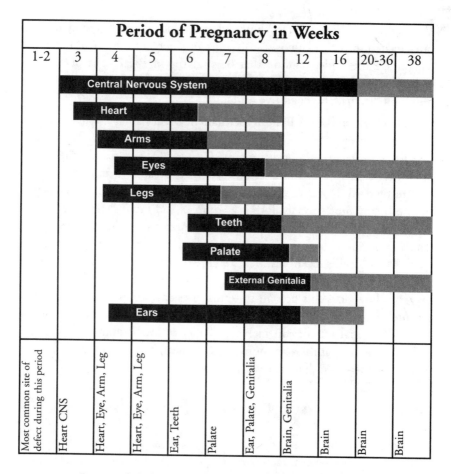

Period of Pregnancy in Weeks

1-2	3	4	5	6	7	8	12	16	20-36	38
Most common site of defect during this period	Heart CNS	Heart, Eye, Arm, Leg	Heart, Eye, Arm, Leg	Ear, Teeth	Palate	Ear, Palate, Genitalia	Brain, Genitalia	Brain	Brain	Brain

Bars: Central Nervous System; Heart; Arms; Eyes; Legs; Teeth; Palate; External Genitalia; Ears

Impact of alcohol use at different points during pregnancy.

The impact of alcohol use during pregnancy is related to such factors as:
1. variations in the timing of alcohol use,
2. variation in the amount of alcohol used,
3. use of more than one substance that can cause birth defects,
4. and many other individual and genetic factors.

The chart above provides an overview of the impact of use at various times over the pregnancy. The dark portion of the bars indicates the most sensitive periods of development, during which the teratogenic effects on the sites listed would result in major structural abnormalities of the child. The lighter portion of the bars shows periods of development during which physiological defects and minor structural abnormalities would occur.

Adapted from Coles, Claire. (1994). "Critical period for Prenatal Exposure." *Alcohol Health and Research World*, 18 (1): 22-29.

Misunderstandings

When these kids act out and it looks like behavior problems, it is a result of permanent, unchanging damage to the brain (static encephalopathy) therefore making the child's behavior out of their control. It is not that they choose not to cooperate, it is that they lack the understanding to do so.

Incurable

FASD cannot be cured, but implementing a structured routine works in helping to maintain the individual's safety. Without early intervention, they have a high risk of developing secondary problems such as conflict with the law, trouble in school and difficulty maintaining successful independence.

Criminalization does not work

An individual living with FASD does not have the ability to navigate through the waters of the criminal justice system. They are incapable of learning from consequence due to brain damage. Their actions are impulsive and without premeditation.

Inability to generalize

Individuals with FASD have an inability to generalize, so when you change a piece of the routine, you have created an entirely new situation and they are seeing it as if for the first time.

People with FASD often look "normal"

It is difficult to look as though you are normal when on the inside there are many difficulties, such as damaged memory, disorganized communication, inability to sequence, inability to generalize information, inability to make connections. Looking normal creates unrealistic expectations.

People with FASD quite often are of normal intelligence

Even though FASD is the leading cause of mental retardation, individuals with this disorder are within a normal IQ range. Whereas people with mental retardation are often affected across the board, individuals with FASD have been found to have areas of great strength and weakness. They can be very gifted in one area while being extremely weak in others.

Teresa Kellerman, an adoptive mother and nationally recognized parent advocate, has written the following song. Teresa's advocacy and a tremendous sense of humor are to be applauded as she continues to be a leader in the world of FASD.

Static Encephalopathy

(sung to the tune of "Supercalifragilisticexpialidocious")

Static encephalopathy, it's really quite atrocious
How everybody's apathy can make us feel ferocious!
Meds or homeopathy might work for some or most of us
But what we need are doctors who can really understand this!

Hum diddle diddle hum diddlie. Hum diddle diddle hum diddlie.

Static encephalopathy, it makes us feel atrocious.
We try to get some sympathy, but what happens to most of us?
Our kids get dropped into the cracks of judicial injustice!
We need a diagnosis quick! Call Drs. Clarren & Streissguth!

Hum diddle diddle hum diddlie. Hum diddle diddle hum diddlie.

Static encephalopathy, the words may sound atrocious.
It means our child will never be the prodigy precocious.
Instead we're seen as parents poor, with judgment they discuss us.
Invisible disabilities that haunt and plague and quash us!

Hum diddle diddle hum diddlie. Hum diddle diddle hum diddlie.

Static encephalopathy makes kids appear atrocious.
So inappropriate they act, they can't control impulses.
But they're just so misunderstood, their little brains can't focus.
The neural pathways just don't work, with overloaded senses.

Hum diddle diddle hum diddlie. Hum diddle diddle hum diddlie.

Static encephalopathy, the term, although atrocious,
Can get the services we need to help our kids, and shows us
That we don't have to suffer from depression and neurosis.
'Cuz static encepalophathy's a worthy diagnosis!

words by Teresa Kellerman 8/22/98

Prevalence Rates

A Health Canada initiative (August, 2000) believes one child a day is born with FAS. It is estimated to be 1-3 per 1000 births in North America (Burgess and Streissguth). The incidence of FAE is about 1 in 300-350. Streissguth goes on to say the statistics are probably very conservative in that they refer to children who have already been identified, referred and diagnosed. This type of birth defect is very hard to measure for a number of reasons. Diagnosis requires confirmation of maternal drinking in pregnancy. A study by Streissguth and Guintal (1988) have found that up to 69% of the biological mothers of FAS children were dead by the time the children reached adolescence and many children are apprehended by Child Welfare, offering no access to biological mothers. Often due to feelings of shame, even when we have access to mom, we do not always receive accurate information regarding her alcohol consumption. This is just one barrier.

How Much is Too Much?

The second is "How much is too much?" Or "How much alcohol is required to cause fetal damage?" This is the question West, a neurobiologist at Texas A&M University of Health Science Centre, researched. The answer was that we do not know due to the fact that alcohol does not have a single threshold as it acts on different biochemical pathways and different parts of the brain. This question about safe amounts of alcohol is difficult to measure and creates a research obstacle, for there is no biological marker to measure alcohol intake and self reports of alcohol consumption may be unreliable, perhaps especially so during pregnancy. It is difficult to measure fetal risk versus alcohol amount. The threshold of alcohol consumption that produces damage is not easy to determine. Based on considerable findings across a large number of studies, research indicates 4-8 drinks a day equals FAS, 2-3 a day equals FAE. Another important variable that comes into consideration is culture and style of drinking and socialization. For example, some cultures would pass around a bottle, therefore it is difficult to measure amount of intake, compared to a culture that drinks where the amount of alcohol consumption can be measured. There are other variables to consider, such as lifestyle, maternal health, nutrition during pregnancy, poverty and its impact on the pregnancy. All of these factors need to be taken into consideration for accuracy in the assessment. A fact that complicates diagnosis efforts further is that infancy is a difficult time to recognize FAS/FAE. Research has not found an amount of alcohol that is safe for the fetus.

New Pattern Emerging

The assumption is often made that babies with FASD are born only to alcoholic mothers. Recent studies have shown this to be not true. Sharon Davies of ARC, a national organization that assists the mentally retarded, has found that the fastest growing group of women giving birth to babies damaged by prenatal alcohol exposure are professional women in their 30s. Researchers agree that a lack of accurate information regarding the pregnancy makes diagnosis more difficult, particularly with FAE. In a recent article in the *Globe and Mail,* they referred to FAS as the silent epidemic among middle class women. It has always been easier to access and study poor women, as they are often on social services or at least accessing community services within inner city communities. The inner city attracts a wealth of studies on poverty, addiction, violence and so on, but the middle class woman is the one that is isolated by her social status, society's expectations and her personal feeling of shaming, self-blaming and responsibility. Although these women often access pre-natal care, the above restrictions may make it more difficult for middle class women to be completely honest.

Binge drinking, for example, is far more common with college students and the white middle class. "Binge drinking is much worse for a developing baby," said Dr. Mary Johnson, a pediatric neurologist. Teresa Kellerman, an expert on FASD, points out that although alcoholic drinking is more common among Native Americans, binge drinking is higher in middle class, white America. Debbie Cohen, director of the New Jersey Office for the Prevention of Mental Retardation and Developmental Disabilities, believes that white children are less likely to be diagnosed. The doctor may not ask about a patient's drinking habits, believing his patients "know better," or that the patient minimizes her use.

Many birth mothers that we have spoken with did not know they were pregnant in the first trimester. We spoke to college girls who were weekend binge drinkers and unaware of risks, thinking weekend drinking was okay. A study from the CDC published in the May 2003 issue of the *Journal of Pediatrics* found that white women who binge drink are more likely to have unintended pregnancies. For 45% of the women in the study, pregnancies were unintended. This study clearly demonstrates that often women don't know that they are pregnant, therefore they are unaware of inflicting fetal harm.

In the course of doing this book, the majority of women that we interviewed were in their late 20s and early 30s. It was surprising – when we asked about their prenatal care, rarely did the women's physicians inquire about their alcohol intake. A number of these women believe that women of poverty have been targeted and identified as being at risk for having children with FASD, but have been led to believe that this is not a personal concern of theirs. The most common question these participants asked was regarding the first trimester and alcohol amounts and the second was the degree of damage caused by a certain amount of alcohol. Both of these questions are excellent and have been posed by scientists and doctors alike, as the desire exists for accurate diagnostic tools for indicating the degree of damage. The important point made here is that FASD is an equal opportunity disorder and it reminds physicians to offer information on FASD to all of their patients, regardless of race or socio-economic class.

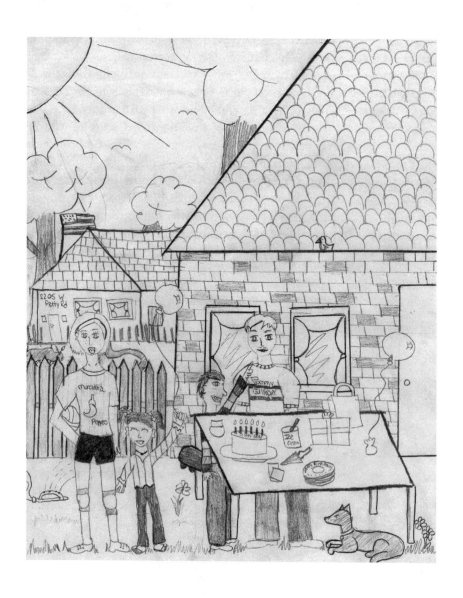

Understanding Behaviors

According to Streissguth (1997), FAS problems are categorized into primary and secondary disabilities. Primary disabilities are a result of brain damage caused by prenatal alcohol exposure, and secondary disabilities are possible consequences of the primary disability. FAS individuals are dealing with learning difficulties such as memory deficits, poor attention span, difficulty in processing information, difficulty with abstract thought, little or no understanding of cause and effect, poor judgement, risk for victimization, difficulty learning from experience, low level problem solving and they will probably need help with basic life skills. Because the children suffer serious damage across a variety of domains, it is the global nature of damage that makes it so disabling for the individual. Children with FAS/FAE often have a superficial facility with language that disguises serious communication problems (Burgess and Streissguth, 1992). There is a general discrepancy between the subjects' ability to use verbal language and the ability to communicate effectively. They have this great superficial conversational talent, but then tend to ignore the messages they receive. It is the secondary disabilities and inability to learn from experiences or understand cause and effect that bring them into conflict with the law.

Secondary disabilities can translate into the behaviors that follow:

1. Easily victimized
2. Unfocused and distractible
3. Difficulty handling money
4. Poor concept of time
5. Trouble learning from experience
6. Problems understanding consequences
7. Poor frustration tolerance
8. Inappropriate sexual behavior
9. Trouble with the law

Taking these into consideration, having FAS/FAE points to the fact that this group will clearly impact on the criminal justice system.

Examples of behaviors as shared by family members

Time

FASD children often have no idea of time and our children were no exception. Often when we were going out, we'd look at the front door and find the girls waiting patiently by the door, with coats, hats and boots on, even if we weren't leaving for an hour. On the other hand, one morning we woke up late and I told the girls we were going to have to "hurry." They had absolutely no idea what I meant and stood totally dumbstruck until I came back later to see why they weren't ready yet. They hadn't even started getting dressed yet since they were still trying to figure out what hurry meant.

How long does it take to go to the washroom at school? At least 45 minutes – 20 minutes to get to the washroom by way of the office, the library, looking out the window, waving at friends in other classes; then 5 or 10 minutes in the washroom itself, checking out all the soap dispensers, toilets, etc., and another 20 minutes following the same route back to the classroom. Just like a scene out of Family Circus!

Eating

It was only days after adopting our sibling group that we realized that eating and table manners were something we were going to have to work on. However we took on this challenge with a vigor that we quickly realized was more than we bargained for. I think that realization came when my birthday supper took us almost 2 hours to eat – well over an hour to eat the main course because we couldn't have dessert until we "cleaned up our plates." My Birthday Cake was finally served after almost an hour and a half at the table.

Our next attempt came at serving the plates away from the table and arranging their food so they would eat their potatoes and vegetables first and meat last. Milk was not served until their plate was clean. That put an end to eating only the meat or gulping down a glass of milk and then claiming to be full. As they grew older, they enjoyed eating enough that this was no longer a challenge, however 2 of my daughters still eat all their potato and vegetables first before savoring the meat last!

Lying

Louise was in ECS when I got the first phone call from school about an incident that had taken place that morning. I chose my moment carefully after the other children were down for their naps so I could quietly discuss the events with Louise. I asked her what had happened at school that morning and then waited patiently while she came up with at least a dozen different versions of the story before she finally looked at me and said "Do you already know?" I was so stunned at her question that I didn't answer and she carried on with half a dozen more versions before finally telling me what had really happened. Creativity at its best!

Giving Instructions

Sometimes my kids just don't get it. We were going away camping in a borrowed motor home for our first vacation with the girls. I spent hours organizing clothes and toys and all the baby paraphernalia required to keep life as "routine" as possible for them. At last we were ready to go and I told them to get in the motor home. We were half way to our destination before I realized that since I had not also told them to put on their shoes, all of them were still wearing their bedroom slippers. Their shoes were all sitting neatly in a row in front of the door at home.

Stealing

It was around 2:00 am when my husband woke up and realized someone was downstairs. As he stood at the top of the stairs, Susan came around the corner. Although she claimed to be getting a drink of water, the dogs were delighted to find out differently. On their way downstairs in the morning, their descent was delayed as they had to stop and eat the pile of cookies Susan had dropped when Dad spotted her during her night time travels.

School

In Grade 1 Sophie was asked to stand at the front of the class and write a math statement as the teacher described it. As she successfully wrote down the problem, the teacher was delighted and very excitely asked her how she got to be so smart in math? Sophie replied – it was because she eats lots of broccoli and it's brain food so it made her smart in Math.

Secondary Disabilities in Teens
– The Slippery Zone

- School drop out or academic failure
- Stealing
- Involvement with crime
- Drug use
- Repetition of behaviors

Inability to Generalize

I once worked with a young girl who worked on the streets as a prostitute. She was the victim of severe sexual assault during which she was taken from the streets and confined. This matter later went to court and a man was convicted of several counts of violence. After the ordeal we talked about the dangers associated with her profession (and discussed ways to keep her safe and prevent violence for her future.)

One day I was doing outreach and I saw this girl across the street from the corner where she was abducted. As I approached her she was very happy and pleased with herself and said, "Look I remembered what you told me about standing on the corner and how dangerous it is for me so I listened and moved to a new corner."

To her, she believed I was referring only to that one physical location, that corner and not the profession of working the streets and standing on the corner engaging in prostitution. She believed she had listened, understood and followed through with my direction and that I would be pleased with her.

Common Sense Valve Broken

"Chicken For Lunch"

A young man named Jeremy was on his way to an interview for a pre-employment program. During the half hour walk downtown he walked through an alley and came across house that had a chicken pen in the back yard. Jeremy then found a cardboard box, began to chase the chickens around the yard, caught one, put it in the box then continued on his way. Arriving late to the interview, he rushed in the office and placed the box on the floor beside his feet.

As the interview got underway, the box started to shake and move across the floor. The program director, stunned, asked the Jeremy what was in the box, "A chicken," Jeremy replied. "Why did you bring a chicken to the interview?" the program director questioned. Jeremy then explained, "I put the chicken in the box so that if I get hungry I can make lunch." Jeremy saw absolutely nothing faulty in his thinking of stealing a chicken and bringing it to the interview.

"Anything Goes"

At 14, Louise first got caught shop-lifting. There was no doubt as the Security Guards witnessed her on camera opening a jar of dill pickles and stuffing a number of them into her mouth before closing up the jar and putting it back on the shelf. Then she moved on to the candy aisle and managed to stuff a bag of chips into her mouth before the security guard arrived on the scene. A search revealed many other items that had been picked up and stuffed into her jacket. When asked why she did it, she said that someone had stolen her lunch at school and she was starving. The security guard verified that she must have been hungry judging by the way she was stuffing all this food into her mouth. On the way home, I asked her where her lunch bag was, to which she replied it was in her backpack. Oops – I guess it wasn't stolen after all! Did she learn not to steal anymore – actually no! What she did learn, though, was not to wear big coats into the store because they'll think you're hiding something and want to search you. Getting caught stealing was nothing, but she really didn't want them searching her.

Individuals with FASD have difficulty translating information from one sense into appropriate behavior, creating gaps in the links.

Poor Judgment

"Adventures in Babysitting"

Samantha, an 18-year-old girl, left her 15-year-old brother, Thomas, to baby-sit her two children while she went to the corner store for diapers and formula. The children were 8 and 22 months old. While she was gone, they began to cry. In an attempt to stop them from crying, Thomas placed a few quilts on top of the babies. When Samantha arrived home 15 minutes later, she found her babies buried under a pile of blankets. Samantha was hysterical and asked her brother what motivated him to do what he did. He then responded, "They were noisy, so I asked them to be quiet, they wouldn't listen so I muffled the sound. I would never hurt them." He believed this and saw nothing *inappropriate with his response to the situation. Following this incident, Samantha came to me with her concerns about her brother's apparent lack of common sense. After discussing her brother's pattern of behavior that stemmed from childhood, we collectively concluded that it was a definite possibility that Thomas had FASD. Diagnostic testing proved that our suspicions were correct. When a worker explained FASD to the girl, she no longer left her brother to baby-sit and encouraged him to get help for FASD.*

Mood Swings

"Living in the Moment"

I was always surprised at how quickly Leanne would trigger mood changes. In fact often I was still considering something she had done or said when she had already forgotten she said anything and moved on. Recently this was witnessed by the Police as well. Things were not going her way and she became quite miserable. As I ignored her behavior, she decided to get my attention. She locked herself in the bathroom and told me she had a knife and was going to cut herself. When this didn't get the desired attention, she told me that if I tried to open the door, it would stick the knife into her back and kill her and I would have to feel guilty for the rest of my life. At that point I decided it was time to put an end to the risk and got Child Welfare and the Police involved, who instructed us to just leave her there until they arrived. My husband and I went outside to wait. The Police arrived within minutes and we escorted them into the house and into the empty bathroom. As the Police officer glanced outside to the yard he spotted Leanne out in the yard laughing and playing with the dog. His only comment to us was, "Is that her? Now I've seen everything. I believe you when you say she's FASD!"

It is important not to jump to conclusions when working with this population, as there can be many misunderstandings. As indicated by these stories the best course of action is to stay calm, communicate, look for appropriate strategies, not take situations at face value and to put in supports if necessary.

Further education and understanding can allow for re-framing of FASD from a negative label to the understanding that it is a lifetime disability. We are not witnessing manipulating, lying, poorly motivated, difficult people, but rather maladaptive behaviors due to neurological impairments.

As we know there has been growth in the area of FASD and there are no easy answers when it comes to providing care to the person affected by FASD. Once the medical profession defined the birth defect, it was the beginning of offering understanding about this sometimes "invisible" and truly complicated disability. There has been a favorable outcome of involvement at many levels. It is heartening to see the judges, corrections officers, lawyers, physicians and clinicians all provide such enlightened recommendations for the problem. It is unfortunate that the wheel of bureaucratic process and change moves so slowly, as it will take time to see those recommendations become a reality.

The community must continue to educate, embrace the recommendations and provide sincere support for the women and their families that we help eliminate the poverty, the drug and alcohol abuse, for a brighter tomorrow for the next generation.

FASD and the Law

It is the cognitive and behavioral problems faced by FAS/FAE individuals that are believed to lead them into trouble with the law. The law, in essence, is based on "cause and effect." Given that FASD individuals are unable to learn from cause and effect, they have an inability to appreciate the impact of the law, therefore punishment will not serve to change their behavior. They did not break the law with intention of a criminal act. Despite the high rates of criminality among FASD individuals, it is important to note that their criminal activities appear largely impulsive rather than premeditated (Streissguth, 1997). She suggests these behaviors arose from maladaptive behaviors and cognitive deficits. Their inability to learn from consequences is what leads them into trouble with the law.

Streissguth, Barr, Kogan and Bookstein (1997) did an important four-year study on secondary disabilities that provides more empirical evidence, suggesting this population is "high risk" for involvement with the criminal justice system. Streissguth collected information from 253 individuals, of which 60% had been in trouble with the law, and of those 50% had been incarcerated. In a study by Fast, Conry and Loocke, all of the youth remanded to a forensic pschiatric in-patient were evaluated over one year and assessed for FASD. Of 287 youth, 23.3% had an alcohol-related diagnosis, 1% had FAS and 22.3% had FAE.

Legal Implications

Many of the behavioral features that are characteristic of FASD have been shown in longitudinal studies to be predictions of delinquency and adult criminal behavior (Farrington, 1995). Recently a report on individuals with FASD (Government of Canada, 1992) gave some recognition to the problems individuals with FASD face with the criminal justice system. Before even beginning the criminal justice process, which includes prosecution, conviction and sentencing, the individual must understand this process, something beyond the scope of the FASD cognitive ability. The judicial system needs to find a more appropriate response to these individuals. FAE is a double-edged sword, for they are more likely to get involved with the criminal justice system because their symptoms go unrecognized, simply because they "look normal." It does not help that they tend to be great conversationalists, without the depth of understanding required for meaningful communication. They also are victims, often willing to "please" others with no appreciation of the consequences, therefore confessing to a crime just to please the person.

Mr. Justice David Vickers, in the case of Victor Daniel Williams, a young man with FAS before the courts, complains that access to support or treatment is available only for those officially labelled. The judge found the state of affairs unsatisfactory, for as we have determined in this book, tools for assessment are few and far between, used mostly for children and not available for the criminal justice system to date. Justice Vickers intended to fashion a sentence for Victor, specific to his individual needs and that would require coordination among agencies. Sentencing is essentially a judicial responsibility, but at the same time, when judges utilize alternative sentencing, they are at the mercy of a functioning bureaucracy whose members do not report to the courts. Justice Vickers speaks to the obvious need to develop innovative interdisciplinary approaches to the custody and treatment of persons whose life circumstances have left them dysfunctional.

Recent research has revealed that our prison system is filled with adults with FAS/FAE. Dr. Christine Loock estimates that at least one in every four inmates in federal institutes has FASD (www. come-over.to/FAS/PrisonersFAS.htm).

Re-framing the situation from an FASD perspective looks something like this:

- failure to appear in court may be due to memory deficit as a result of brain damage
- not going to probation appointment could be a situation of becoming distracted on the way to the appointments and then
- forgetting where you are going
- a confession just to please an authority figure
- changing what he/she said could be confusion rather than lying
- repeating back what was said to them should not indicate a level of comprehension

As we view the criminal justice process with the knowledge of what it is to have FASD, a new picture is painted of a person with organic brain damage who is trying to make sense of this criminal justice process as best he is able and is still coming up short.

FASD – A Serious Reality:
Interview with Cathy Lane Goodfellow

Here is the question posed: "If a person with FASD commits a horrific crime, should criminal sanctions be applied? Why or why not?" Consider the case of David Trott, a young man who pled guilty to the brutal rape and murder of nine-year-old Jessica Russell in Mission B.C. (http://www.canoe.ca/NationalTicker/CANOE-wire.CRIME-Trott.html). During his childhood and adolescence, Trott had been shuffled through more than 50 foster homes following the death of his mother. Trott has been diagnosed with numerous behavioral problems, one of which is FASD. The trial was delayed a year due to the fact that Trott was not found mentally fit to stand trial. There is no question that David Trott committed this crime and there is no question that the brutality of this crime warrants harsh punishment. What remains in question is what measures must be taken to provide appropriate sentencing to satisfy both the needs of the convicted with disabilities and the safety of the community.

First, let us review how FASD could have contributed to this crime. We will review what we know to be true. A person with FASD, such as David Trott, often acts on impulse, is unable to understand cause and effect, attaches no meaning to consequences and is unable to learn from experience.

Next we look at sentencing objectives in accordance with the Criminal Code of Canada:

1. To denounce unlawful conduct.

2. To detour the offender and other persons from committing offences.

3. To separate offenders from society when necessary.

4. To assist in rehabilitating an offender.

5. To provide reparations for harm done to victims or the community.

6. To promote a sense of responsibility in offenders and the acknowledgment of harm to victims and the community.

Let us look again at the situation. If these are the objectives of sentencing, then due to the nature of the disorder, an individual with FASD will never be detoured by jail because consequences are meaningless and do not impact their behavior. Jail is also counterproductive, as it separates them from society and places them in an environment where they will be victimized and learn how to become better criminals. Rehabilitation would require a special program that understands their behaviors and needs – such programs are rare and the few that exist cannot keep up with the demand. To promote responsibility is not possible for the crimes were impulsive, could happen again and probably will.

The situation is by no means simple; neither are the solutions. Chances are good that the criminal with FASD will re-offend. Options in sentencing are difficult to apply given the reality of FASD and the question remains how will justice be served. How do we effectively support this person, who is both victim of circumstances and a perpetrator of criminal activity?

In an interview with Cathy Lane Goodfellow, an attorney specializing in youth criminal defence, we explored two areas of concern regarding individuals with FASD who are before the courts.

The first area that we explored was the amount of education law students received regarding FASD and how this disability impacts representing their clients. Cathy spoke of the benefits of a recent conference on FASD tailored to the needs of the legal community and spearheaded by Judge Cookstan Hope. The two-day conference presented a wealth of information and left Cathy with a new understanding that was beneficial to working with individuals with FASD. In this conference they learned about the secondary disabilities, the diagnosis process, heard from birth mothers and about funding to gain help in the law community. Cathy said at the end of the day, you can have the knowledge about FASD, but it is the application that is important in regards to the law. "We gained the knowledge but are not sure how to apply it. If criminal sanctions are not imposed on criminals, what are we supposed to do? We rely on the criminal justice system to handle the juveniles who can not be handled by child welfare and social services. People need to know and understand how serious FASD is." Cathy recalled a case in which a young man was charged with beating an older man to death with a bat. He had clear symptoms of FASD – by the second day in jail he did not understand why he was there. He was 16 years old and was tried in youth court; if he was found not criminally responsible, he would then go into the hospital system. This is not an issue that can be white washed or cast as a Native issue and dismissed, it cannot be ignored. Addressing the legal implications of FASD is a social responsibility that needs to be addressed.

We have to get society to believe that children are in need of protection. Common opinion has not completely aligned with this view; many think that adolescents are responsible for their behavior and should be locked up like anyone else. Everything related to children, especially adolescents in this province, is in crisis, the education system, child welfare, youth corrections.

The second area of concern is the need to change our attitude, for it is really unfair to blame, you have to forgive the mother, it is not always about women who can't cope with parenting. Sometimes it is better to leave the child with the mother to heal the family for the betterment of the child, the family and in the long run our entire community. In law school you do not learn how to handle children, no information on adolescent development is part of the curriculum, which is not fair to the future lawyers and the clients that they will represent.

We do not value children and we are afraid of adolescents.

For a lot of lawyers it is not about understanding the child, it is about whether or not they did the crime, it is about leading them in and out of the system, that's it. It is a common dynamic. You are rarely going to find a law professor that will consider advocating for their client as part of their job description, they do not want to be social workers to their clients.

I worry about the future of youth criminal law, especially legal aid, who are often the representing agents of these clients. How do we convince young lawyers that this is a good job?

I have memories of certain children that I have represented over the years, it is the memory of these children who we have failed that encourages me to continue doing the work that I do.

The Several Languages of Law

By David Boulding

I BELIEVE that the various people who work in the criminal legal system often speak in a technical way using words that persons not trained in law find confusing and hard to understand. This technical use of language makes it difficult for parents and caregivers of persons with Fetal Alcohol Syndrome (FAS) to communicate with the several parts of the criminal law system. Sometimes the criminal legal system stoops to using Latin words like *actus reus* or *mens rea* or gets weird with its words, using complicated sentences like the ones found in probation orders. These unusual styles of language often mystify listeners without legal experience.

I believe it is possible to translate criminal legal language into plain English by examining the role of each speaker and then isolating the language unique to that speaker: police speak differently about your son than do doctors who are trained to assess children who might have FAS.

As a parent/caregiver to a person with FAS, you can learn to hear the different languages of law. I offer here a few hints that might be helpful to you.

My assumptions are:

1. I assume that all workers in the criminal legal system are honorable folks trying to do the best they can given what they know about FAS.

2. I assume that each person or department of the criminal legal system may conflict with other persons or departments in the criminal legal system because many people know very little about FAS.

3. I am stating here my opinions which are based on 15 years in the criminal legal system. I am assuming others will have different ideas. These comments are suggested as a guide for parents and caregivers of persons with FAS. My words are not legal advice. I urge listeners/readers to meet a defence counsel, a lawyer who specializes in defending persons accused of crimes. It is vital to your child's future that as caregivers you have a positive relationship with your defence lawyer – whether the lawyer be from legal aid or one you have hired privately.

4. I assume you know lawyers cost money. There are ways to lower the cost: the Canadian Bar Association Lawyer Referral System, legal aid, the pro bono system also from the Canadian Bar and the UBC student lawyers (LSLAP). I believe a criminal defence lawyer is as important to your child's future as is Doctor Asante and Doctor Conry. This may sound trivial to you. It is true for me: I have never regretted paying Bill Gopaul, my mechanic, the thousands of dollars I have paid him in the last 10 years to keep my truck on the road and safe. Thus I assume your child is more important to you than my 1990 Ford 4x4 F 250 truck is to me.

5. My last assumption is my strongest belief: **If We Knew How the Brain Really Worked We Would Punish Differently.** This means we must educate ourselves and all members of the criminal legal system about FAS. And this education process will be our life's work.

The several languages of law are spoken by judges, police, probation officers, prison guards, crown counsel, defence counsel, social workers, psychologists, doctors, forensic workers and courthouse librarians. All of these legal workers have different roles and duties. Because they all have a different focus, they speak differently about the FAS person as the FAS person navigates the criminal legal system.

And because each person has a different understanding of FAS, these people and their opinions and the words they use conflict with each other, often to the detriment of the person with FAS.

Police

They are the receptionists for the criminal legal system…the point of first contact. Police speak of detection: they ask "WHO DUNNIT?"

Police speak as investigators, gathering facts so they can write a report to Crown Counsel saying your child stole the car, left his fingerprints on the mirror and did 3900 dollars in damage…he had no permission to be in the car owned by Mrs. Smith of 2003 Granville. You have heard Sergeant Friday say: "just the facts ma'am."

Police have some discretion, often more than anyone else in the system, so it is tempting for parents to speak to police in a parent to parent language. This is a mistake in 99.99% of the cases. Police do not hear "permanent brain damage" as satisfactory language. Police will say "theft is an offence, your son did it and I have the necessary proof, therefore my role in this case is closed." If they do hear the parent speak about FAS, police will think that FAS is a type of problem that is in the "not in their department" category. Police believe that FAS as an explanation for criminal conduct is something for the doctors in jail to sort out.

Caution Caution Caution Caution Caution

Most people are convicted on the evidence they give to police, often thinking that they can explain their way out of trouble by talking to the nice policeman…this is doubly true in youth court. Parents often make the same mistake. Some parents help the police because they are exhausted and can no longer "handle" the FAS child… these parents may think that a break for them and some time in jail for their son will be in the best interests of their child…so they speak to police in a parent to parent voice using the common language of caring parents. While on the job, police are not parents… they hear "he dunnit" and they stop listening because their job is finished.

This means that parents must learn to say to police:

"MY SON NEEDS A LAWYER NOW. MY SON DOES NOT WAIVE HIS RIGHT TO SILENCE. HE IS ASSERTING HIS

RIGHT TO COUNSEL AS GUARANTEED IN THE CHARTER OF RIGHTS AND FREEDOMS."

Parents need to understand that rarely (often never) does it assist your son to help police with their investigations. Your wish for a lawyer does not mean you are assisting in criminal conduct, nor does it mean you must behave in a boorish, obnoxious way.

Be clear! Your son's interests and the police's interests are not the same....Jail will not help a person with FAS. Give your son the same legal rights and the same access to legal services that a successful West Vancouver business man takes for granted: get a lawyer.

Curb your natural desire to explain your love for your son and provide examples of his good behavior...transform that energy into a simple phone call to a professional who is skilled at dealing with police questions.

Crown Counsel, Crown Attorneys and Crown Prosecutors

They are public servants who behave according to the highest standard of public behavior. They are not your lawyer: they are lawyers to and for the province of British Columbia.

They do not win or lose cases.

They stand up in court and do the right thing as might be defined by an impartial fair witness from your community. This fairness obligation is a legal requirement that each Crown takes seriously.

Although Crowns speak about fairness, they also speak about the victim's pain and loss and will list in great detail the hurts suffered by a victim and will often ignore the hurt suffered by the accused FAS person.

Crowns speak in two styles – in court voice – designed to persuade a judge to see the case from the Crown's eyes – and in an out of court voice – a voice of a normal person you might meet on the street.

Do Not Confuse the Out of Court Crown Who is a Pleasant Person with the Tough Lawyer You Hear in Court.

They have these different voices, different languages, for different reasons. Crowns often have to do fact gathering. So as a fact collector interviewing you as a parent, the Crown will present as a compassionate listener. Understand that when a Crown prosecutor speaks to you out of court, he is like a policeman gathering facts to secure a conviction, so the caution about police applies to Crown attorneys also. Let your defence counsel lawyer do the talking to Crown for the same reasons you must not talk to police.

When in court, Crown counsels speak about criminal rules and evidence as proof. Often parents will speak to a Crown out of court and give facts to the Crown that prove the guilt of the FAS person. Again and again, parents are surprised that the Crown "twisted their words" when the parent was only trying to explain how their son really is. This mistake is made by parents because they do not recognize the language of a prosecutor. I believe prosecutors never lie, while police will often misstate or exaggerate and sometimes lie.

The consequences for a Crown lying are drastic... boom bang and they are no longer a lawyer. Parents may think the prosecutor is not telling the truth. I believe parents mean the Crown is not telling the whole story as the parent sees the truth. This is a critical point: a Crown must be fair, while not obligated to tell the whole story as you the caregiver sees it.

Our criminal legal system is an adversarial process – lawyers fight and argue about what really happened – and a judge decides. This means Crown tells one side – usually the police side – and your defence counsel tells another side of the story.

Parents who listen to the Crown often hear only the police side of what happened and believe the Crown is being unfair. **No, Absolutely Not True!**

As a parent you are hearing the language of a lawyer seeking a conviction based on the evidence collected by the Crown from police. In a trial your lawyer, the defence, will get his turn: much of the criminal legal system is about waiting.

Criminal cases in British Columbia go to court only if two questions are answered with "yes."

Is there a reasonable likelihood of conviction?

Is it in the public interest to proceed?

From these questions you can see that Crowns speak in a language of proof and then in a language of what is the public good. The first is specific information gathered by the police, the second is a language of philosophy of what is good for all citizens. In these questions, there appears no specific place or spot for persons with FAS. The first is a technical question. It is legalistic in language. The second question is about what kind of community do we want to live in. It is in the second question, before charges are laid, that your defence counsel can sometimes work for your son. Here you have input. Your lawyer can try to persuade the charge approval Crown to not criminalize the mentally incompetent, or discriminate against people with permanent brain damage, or warehouse the mentally compromised.

At the **sentencing** part of the trial, Crowns speak about punishment. Here the Crown will emphasize again the hurt of the victim and will use victim impact statements that are often recited in the inflammatory language of victims. Crown counsel will emphasize the criminal record of your son and likely suggest jail, because as Crown they will say "jail will protect the public and protect the reputation of the criminal legal system." When you listen to Crown at the sentencing stage, often you will not recognize your son because the Crown is speaking in a language of persuasion, trying to convince the judge to put your son in jail. Your lawyer will get his turn: again you must wait.

Defence Lawyers, Defence Counsel and Legal Aid Lawyers

These are the hired guns of the legal system. Defence counsel is your champion in this legal fight, disguised as your son's court case. Defence counsel speaks specifically to your son, not you, they take instruction from your son, not you. Defence counsels are also driven by facts and they are most interested in your son's personal facts. Here then is the one person you can talk to without any filters, without any editing, without caution....you can open your heart to defence counsel because she can use those facts you give her when speaking to a judge.

Because defence counsel are single minded – they aim to shoot Crown and their Crown facts until the Crown cases dies – often defence counsel will say to parents while in court: "I don't need to know that now. Write it down for me." So take the time required and write down in clear English what you believe your son's lawyer needs to know. When your lawyer says the above, she means she is busy and is thinking about something important or she may mean she does not understand what makes the comment you have important to the case.

That sort of comment should ring bells in you. If it is important to you it must be important to defence counsel – you may have to re-frame your words to defence counsel so your words can assist in getting a not guilty decision or help convince the judge to give a punishment of fewer months in jail.

Probation Officers

These overworked people speak of compliance: they demand compliance because they are paid to make sure your son follows the court order. Their language is full of "must" and "should" words. They believe that by following court orders your son will not re-offend and will change his behavior – they are strict sorts of people and believe in simple carrot and the stick psychology…in 15 years I have not met a probation officer I did not like. As a rule the ones who deal with kids or mentally disordered offenders really do care. And as parents you will hear caring in their words. Remember they are police officers: they can issue breach charges by a phone call….when they say comply they mean: "do as I say or go to jail."

Obviously few probation officers use the heavy hand of jail all the time. Next to defence counsel, the probation officer often speaks in a language recognized by parents. Probation officers are court appointed parents and parents will do well to have the best relationship possible with the probation office. "On time each time" and "do it my way" are words probation often use to secure compliance.

Probation officers are most likely the only person in the system open to negotiation with parents. Probation officers will get more flexible as your son follows the orders. In this way you can see that probation officers are much like parents.

Provincial Court Judges

Provincial court judges are the workhorses of the criminal legal system.

They have seen everything you can imagine, often three times a day.

Judges speak two distinct languages.

1. The language of proof and of rules and of admissible evidence and of beyond a reasonable doubt – this is the technical legal language of law.

2. The language of punishment: at sentencing where the judge decides the punishment for your son.

This second language is clearly set out in the criminal code in *Part XXIII, Sentencing: Section 716 to Section 751.* Codes are available in courthouse libraries.

According to the Criminal Code, Judges Must Do the Following:

1. Protect the public.

2. Denounce unlawful conduct.

3. Jail people if necessary.

4. Assist in rehabilitation.

5. Provide for the harm done to victims.

6. Promote responsibility in offenders.

7. Acknowledge harm to victims.

Rehabilitation is the Biggest Hope of Every Judge.

Many judges believe that rehabilitation is the best way to protect the public.

In their first language style during the trial, judges speak of guilty or not guilty. Thus judges speak about complex criminal rules of procedure. It is only in the second part of the trial, in the sentencing stage, when judges speak in a language about punishment, that as a parent you must listen carefully. This language is almost always plain English because then the judge is speaking directly to you and your son.

During the second part of the trial called "speaking to sentence," where the judge speaks the language of punishment, you can have the most impact as a parent. Here the defence lawyer is allowed to let you, your doctor or any other person speak to the judge. If some one has something to say that can help your son's case, here the judge will relax the strict rules of criminal procedure and listen.

Here the judge will speak to your son and to you in a way much like a conversation before the judge makes a decision on what is the appropriate punishment.

Here your son – as a person in a community – is the only topic. As a member of a community your son has caused harm and the judge must decide how to protect the community and assist your son in not making the same mistake. I believe at the sentencing is where good lawyers shine and lazy lawyers do a disservice to their clients and the reputation of the criminal legal system.

Judges are professional listeners: they are consumers of evidence. It is at the sentencing stage where you can best speak to the judge and assist the judge in understanding fetal alcohol syndrome.

Much Like a Parent, the Judge is Trying to Change Behavior While Protecting Your Community.

At Sentencing, You Must Insist on a Complete Fetal Alcohol Syndrome Assessment by Experts.

You may be able to get an assessment ordered by the judge, at the first appearance, if your son's lawyer can convince the judge there is an issue of "fitness to stand trial." This means the lawyer will tell the judge as a lawyer he has concerns his client may not be fit to stand trial without a complete FAS assessment from an expert. If you already have an assessment and diagnosis, give the report to the defence counsel the first time you meet your son's lawyer. Note that assessments are hard to obtain unless you can pay the $2500 to $3000 each costs.

Legal System Helpers

Social workers, forensic staff, most psychologists, psychiatrists and family doctors can be grouped together as legal system helpers. They advise judges and lawyers with their specific expert knowledge. If they have expert knowledge, they are helpful. Obviously as parents you know that these good folks often know nothing about FAS because they are trapped by the book of official mental illnesses called the DSM, which does not list FAS as an "official mental disease."

Here you will hear either:

1. I don't know ANYTHING about FETAL ALCOHOL SYNDROME
   Or

2. you will hear words like: ADHD, oppositional defiant disorder, conduct disorder, anti-social disorder, learning disability disorder, lack of impulse control, refusal to comply, poor choices, lack of executive decision-making, poor time management, few financial skills and similar piecemeal descriptions of behavior.

As you know, you will not hear that your son has permanent brain damage caused in the womb by alcohol consumption by the mother.

To find knowledgeable professionals, contact the Asante Centre, the FAS Network, or your local Children's Hospital.

Beautiful Librarians:
The Goddesses of Legal Knowledge

The last and most important people in the criminal legal system are the Law Librarians.

Unlike anyone else in the legal system, librarians speak plain English and can show you between the hours of 9 am and 4 pm where all the law books are hidden that may assist you.

They can show you how to use your home computer to find similar cases like yours. They can tell you what judges are learning when they go to judge school and they can show you the criminal codes and all kinds of wonderful materials that can help you communicate with the different and conflicting parts of the criminal legal system.

Lawyers and judges depend on librarians, because no one person can know everything about law except a talented law librarian. They are lifesavers; I speak from experience. There is not a lawyer alive who has not been saved by a law librarian: I know I am one of the saved.

The best thing: they are free.

Conclusion

Perhaps now you can begin to understand the different languages of law and how you can communicate with the different and conflicting aspects of the criminal law system.

My main suggestion is that you as a parent/caregiver find a criminal lawyer you like and trust and develop a professional relationship with a criminal defence lawyer identical to the one you and your son have with your doctor.

My next suggestion is going to cause a fuss and I think it is worth talking about today especially with parents/caregivers of persons with FAS here today.

Perhaps your son/daughter should carry a laminated photo identification card like your driver's licence that states:

1. Your child's name, address and phone number of parent/caregiver.
2. That this pictured person has permanent brain damage – as a result of a birth defect.
3. That the brain damage this pictured person has may be a factor in a list of negative behaviors.
4. This pictured person insists on speaking to a lawyer if arrested or detained by anyone including police.
5. This pictured person does not waive his right to silence.
6. This pictured person is asserting all his charter rights immediately upon arrest or detention by any person including the police.
7. Please call the criminal defence lawyer listed below or arrange for the police to call emergency defence counsel on the telephone immediately.

Note: the Brydges lawyer is a lawyer paid by legal aid to answer a telephone 24 hours a day, 7 days a week to answer questions free – that means

MEDICAL INFORMATION FOR POLICE

I have the birth defect Fetal Alcohol Spectrum Disorders (FASD), which causes brain damage. If I need assistance, or if you need my cooperation, you should contact the person listed on the back of this card.

Because of this birth defect, I do not understand abstract concepts like legal rights. I could be persuaded to admit to acts that I did not actually commit. I am unable to knowingly waive any of my constitutional rights, including my right to counsel.

Because of my disability, I do not wish to talk with law enforcement officials except in the presence of and after consulting with an attorney. I do not consent to any search of my person or property.

For information or assistance regarding:

Please contact:

Doctor or diagnostician:

For information about FASD call Joining Forces—Fetal Alcohol Society (403) 202-7233

The above card (shown back and front) was created by Joining Forces. Rather than providing a photo, they require listing the FASD person's physician as a contact for identification.

at no cost to the caller – to persons who cannot contact their own defence lawyer when arrested by the police.

This card maybe called a Medical Information Card for Police. The reason a picture is required is to prevent other criminals from using FAS as an excuse to commit crimes and try to get away with it. I suspect this may sound like a futuristic police state kind of response to many here. I am told that in Quebec, developmental disability advocates are beginning to use similar cards.

Future Recommendations

We have seen from Justice Vickers' attempt at sentencing without a label or diagnosis, how difficult it could be. Streissguth (1997) has outlined a number of potential benefits of diagnosis:

1. Promotes visibility in order to offer help

2. Identifies a cause, therefore encouraging understanding, education and realistic goals

3. Motivates appropriate treatment, intervention and identifies and acknowledges those suffering from FAS

4. Diagnosis records can aid in further research or needs assessments and recidivism

Streissguth also argues that a tracking system for FAS across multiple agencies would greatly improve the services for these individuals.

Two tools used for screening are FABS, Fetal Alcohol Behavior Scale (FABS: Streissguth, Barr and Press, 1996). This measures typical behavior. Second "the LHI" (Life History Interview) (LHI: Streissguth, Barr, Kogan, Bookstein, 1997). This is used to study many secondary disabilities across a life span.

One of the major current needs is to develop a standardized screening procedure; researchers and clinicians have yet to formally agree on a diagnostic assessment tool.

Judicial education is an important factor in developing alternative strategies for persons with intellectual, emotional or physical disabilities.

The society could support innovative new approaches such as the Triumf Project, which takes the weaknesses of FAS and turns them into strengths.

In addressing innovative approaches, we could start with the police, who, when they discover an intoxicated pregnant woman, should offer her supports to social services.

We, as a community, must attempt to help, not to blame, for we live in a society where drinking alcohol is encouraged, easily available, often glamorized and then it is taboo for a pregnant woman.

Crime

Persons with FASD often re-offend upon release

Accurate assessments can have tremendous implications for how the criminal justice system handles the FASD individuals. One law professor goes on to say, "It is analogous to the mental disorder defense in the sense that we've said that people who are affected should not be punished in the usual criminal justice sense." FASD is not an excuse for one's actions, rather how can we utilize punishment when the person does not understand what they have done wrong and more importantly, if they cannot comprehend the concept of consequences due to the disorder.

We must also bear in mind that many FASD individuals live in the moment, very much in the present, and are forgetful of rules and like to please others. So in essence we have an individual who is going to tell you what you want to hear, without the understanding that he is compromising himself by telling things that are untrue and implicating him in crimes. Actually the FASD person might feel happy simply because the other person seems pleased, not seeing the bigger picture that they are under arrest.

With these realities, it is not hard to understand just how the FASD individual can come into conflict with the law. Once in jail they do well, seem to adjust and do not misbehave until out of the structured environment where temptation is back in the picture. We already have high risk factors when we house an individual with FASD who is impressionable, demonstrates poor boundaries and immaturity, and is housed with hardened criminals where they could be taught bad behaviors. At best we can say they are surrounded by poor role models and in reality they are in an environment where they can easily fall victim to physical and sexual assaults, given the milieu.

Our system fails the FASD person because we know consequences don't work, punishment is ineffective and not deterrent. We also know that protection is imperative, and structure is beneficial. An appropriate rehabilitation program would be beneficial. Incarcerating the FASD individual is to do these individuals a great disservice at the hand of justice.

FASD individuals have a difficult if not impossible task advocating for themselves before our justice system. The legal waters are too complicated for the FASD individuals to navigate without help. The outcome is not productive if they go to jail and have the quality of their lives impacted so negatively.

A potentially difficult area for the courts is that the FASD individual can know the rules, even know the consequences. Yet this is irrelevant, for they are unable to follow through with the appropriate actions. They repeat the same mistakes over and over and over. Their challenge lies in trying to do what they are supposed to do based on knowledge of both the rules and consequences. Yet here is when the problem exists: they have an inability to learn from past experiences, lack an awareness of consequences or cannot predict outcome. For the individual with FASD, they may repeat the same offence as if it is for the first time. The first 50 times I saw this behavior, I was amazed to see such a lack of awareness. Now it is predictable because I understand how the disorder presents itself. What was once invisible for me is now visible.

There is a difficult zone for parents, a gray zone, as many teenagers may hit upon one of these categories as normal acting out. The FASD teenagers will present these behaviors with the key of repetition as an indicator of grave concern. They repeat the problem endlessly. There was one young man I worked with who spent the majority of his life from 12 to 24 years behind bars. He is a sweet and gentle boy who would repeat two offences, car theft and general theft. The amazing fact about this young man was that he was often charged with a new crime within a week of his release from jail. I worked with his sister and family members to offer support, yet without educating the family about the young man's FASD the family saw his behavior as intentional and they were angry at him and worn out with the sheer number of offences. With education and understanding for the family, they were able to deal with their frustrations in a more productive manner.

I would like to introduce a letter by a lawyer in Vancouver speaking to his experience working with clients with FASD.

Mistakes That I Have Made with FAS Clients

by David Boulding

My remarks are tentative and personal. There are probably more mistakes I have made and perhaps I am unaware of them or I choose to remain unaware.

It Is Embarrassing to Admit

It is embarrassing to admit my mistakes. I encourage you to tell me what your experience has been with lawyers' mistakes, because you can help me learn even more.

My intention here is not just to confess, although this paper clearly is a confession by one lawyer who believes that the Canadian legal system has failed FAS clients. I hope to show in this article that there is hope. We can change how lawyers, clients, police, judges, probation officers, prison guards and family members work with FAS clients.

The List of My Mistakes as a Lawyer

1. I assumed that both my young offender FAS clients and my adult FAS clients could be helped by using standard terms of Probation Orders in the Provincial Court.

2. I assumed that my FAS clients could tell the Judge what happened in a way that would make sense.

3. I assumed that my FAS clients would be able to demonstrate remorse to the Sentencing Judge.

4. I assumed that after my clients were caught for the third or fourth time for the same offence and in the same set of circumstances, that at least they would learn to get caught for either another offence, wear gloves, or not be surprised that they were caught.

5. I assumed that my FAS clients understood the notion of consequences: if you steal from cars and are caught, you will go to jail.

6. I assumed that my FAS clients understood the notion of time – three days in jail is not the same as three months in jail.

7. I failed to tell my FAS clients the same important lawyer/client advice over and over again. Perhaps I should have handed my FAS clients a typed handout setting out what a guilty plea means and the specific short and long term consequences. I assumed that because we had been to Court many times, that my clients would know that they should not interrupt the Crown Prosecutor during a "Show Cause Hearing," correct the Crown Prosecutor's facts and therefore admit that they were there and that they did it.

8. Although I knew the parents of my clients, I failed to discuss with the parents the apparently "crazy" situation. I knew that the parents had had severe drinking problems for years, but I never asked anyone about

the home life and I never asked my client about his/her parents' drinking. I never directly confronted the parents about maternal drinking during pregnancy.

9. I was always puzzled and failed to understand that there is a good reason why, in the Pre-Sentence Reports of the Probation Officers, my FAS clients seemed to "shoot themselves in the foot." My FAS clients participated completely and without guile in their Pre-Sentence Reports. I failed to understand that the reason they were so candid, up front, and straight with the Probation Officers was that they did not know how to play the "Pre-Sentence Report" game. My FAS clients were impressionable, suggestible and easily mislead and misunderstood. It was easy for the Probation Officers to get them to give the answers that the Crown oriented Probation Officers wanted. My FAS clients did not understand the vocabulary that lawyers, judges and probation officers use everyday. My FAS clients were eager to please. I failed to see that they were speaking against their own interests. A common example was a client's admitting to either drug or alcohol use, but failing to mention frequency or context.

10. I failed to consider that there were some offences, in some situations, where I should have considered a *Not Criminally Responsible By Reason of a Mental Disease* (NCRMD) application. At least I might have begun to gather some neuro-psychological data years ago.

11. I failed to consider breaches of the Canadian Charter of Rights and Freedoms, although I found that most Crown Prosecutors were helpful in reducing the number of the charges. Often there were 13 or 14 separate counts. I never noticed that my clients had long Criminal Records and almost always pleaded guilty. I did not realize that there was a behavior problem at the brain level. I failed to look past the standard phrase "anti-social disorder." I failed to see that my clients were not learning by experience and that a Charter breach from Section 15 Equality Before the Law was something I should have considered. These clients were not being treated equally and the system had failed to accommodate their special needs. A brain injury by definition makes you a "special needs" person. FAS clients suffer a lifetime of brain injury inflicted by a mother who drank alcohol during prenatal fetal development.

12. I failed to consider a psychological or neurological assessment at any time because my clients seemed so pleasant. My clients did not seem to have any outward signs of psychological difficulties. They did not

have any drug or alcohol problems. I failed to consider that there might be something wrong with their brain.

13. I failed to see that behind my clients' cheery, positive presentation of self lurked another problem. To most judges, police officers, probation people, and other lawyers, my clients did not present themselves as really bad kids. My clients tended to present themselves as first-time offenders who had made some silly one-time "mistake." The problem was they actually had long Criminal Records for those same "mistakes."

14. I failed to ask Social Services for records about the family. I never looked at any early medical records for my clients. I never considered looking at any medical records.

15. I failed to note that my FAS clients were usually the number two or number three person involved in the offense, but that it was always my FAS clients that were caught. I did not recognize that there must be a reason that other people initiated the offences and were rarely arrested while my clients were always caught.

16. I failed to see that there was no real escalation in the offenses. The marijuana-to-heroin jump never happened. The auto theft-to-robbing jewelry stores jump never happened. I failed to see that this lack of escalation indicated the lack of a professional criminal element or what I call "real criminality," characterized by mean, nasty, and cruel behavior. I believe the offenses involved an absolute moment-by-moment "I want, I take" mechanism as opposed to some deeply ingrained refusal to follow rules. My FAS clients did not present as outlaws, but as serial opportunistic criminals – repeaters of first-time offender behavior.

17. I failed to notice that when my clients were telling their story, there were blanks in their memories or parts of the story were just not available. My clients did not remember important facts. My clients did not know the answers to some of my "and then what?" questions. I failed to take detailed written instructions for the offenses because they were so similar and were almost always repetitions of the same facts. Had I asked the clients to write out, in detail, what happened, I might have eventually seen the need for neurological help.

18. I failed to understand the nature of my clients' impulsive activity because they told their stories in an amusing and funny way to both the police officers and me. I failed to look past the clients' rather humorous and engaging presentation of self.

19. I failed to get written instructions and keep a running file on my Fetal Alcohol Syndrome clients' criminal activity. If I had sat down with them and had them write out their instructions, I *might* have seen a chance or found some way of getting the message "Don't do this again" to sink in. Nevertheless, I may still be in denial in terms of not understanding the scope of the brain injury. I failed to see that my clients did not understand while they were doing it, that stealing from cars is wrong.

20. I failed to see that jail had no effect on my clients' behavior. The main reason they didn't want to go to jail was that they couldn't be with their friends. If they did go to jail with friends, the experience did not seem to have any impact. On two occasions, one FAS client escaped with his cousin; my client was caught – his cousin remained at large for months.

21. I failed to talk to other lawyers and other probation officers about the particular set of facts that kept reappearing.

22. I never asked one of my FAS clients' mothers directly about alcohol consumption, perhaps out of some sort of misinformed political correctness or perhaps because I was too shy. I didn't want to embarrass the mothers, as many of these women were aboriginal women, who clearly had too many difficulties to begin with. I never asked about alcohol consumption patterns in the home. Quite often, these mothers were in tears when their sons were in jail. I simply did not fully understand the family circumstances.

23. Although I acted for most of the family members, I never sat down and drew out a family tree and tried to figure out who was who and what family member had what particular problem. I never put into place structures that would help my client with follow-through, such as giving the Probation Officer the telephone number of the most dependable relative or putting into place some type of back-up or support system to check on the client in an ongoing way.

24. My FAS clients often did not follow through with basics, like showing up for appointments, being on time, going to the right places, or conducting themselves appropriately. I tried to simplify Probation Orders to make it as easy as possible because I thought my client just could not handle complex orders. My assumption that my clients were not interested or did not care was wrong: they could not structure the pieces of the puzzle together in a logical and meaningful way.

25. I did not understand that this inability to handle complex notions of responsibility and consequences was something I needed to consider. I should have asked myself, "Is he getting a fair trial?" I failed to ask, "Why all the guilty pleas?" I failed to consider "fitness for trial," because to the outside world, they seemed okay. For example, although one client had only an eighth-grade education, he played basketball, and he seemed to be one of those kids who just did not like school. I failed to look at the whole person in the context of Fetal Alcohol Syndrome and criminal Courts.

26. I failed to sit down and write out all of the various excuses my FAS clients gave for the various offences. Had I taken the time to write down and study the 10 or 15 excuses, I would have recognized the need for professional help. Instead, I kept treating each offense in isolation, not understanding that it was the same crazy offense over and over again, with outlandish rationalizations, or simple-minded explanations.

27. I failed to see that often within the aboriginal community, aunts distantly related to my FAS clients understood there was a problem and instinctively took care of my clients for various periods of their lives. It was during those periods of intense supervision that my FAS clients were crime-free. However, as soon as that supervision went away, leaving my clients alone, it was predictable that they would return to familiar criminal behavior.

28. I did not notice that constant supervision by an appropriate parental authority corresponded to a lack of crime. I never understood that there was an impulse control problem, even though almost all of the crimes were related to acquiring household goods or getting immediate pleasures, as opposed to crime requiring any sophisticated planning or violence. There were, of course, some exceptions.

29. I failed to see that my clients were not competent thieves. They did not plan. They were opportunistic and impulsive. For example one client spent ten minutes breaking into a car, while being observed by the police.

The Biggest Mistake

The biggest mistake I have made as a lawyer regarding dealing with clients who suffer from Fetal Alcohol Syndrome was my lack of political awareness.

I am now aware that the list of my mistakes is going to cost my clients time – time spent in jail. My clients are paying for my mistakes.

It is my opinion that the Government of British Columbia is complicit in my clients' criminalization. The British Columbia Government is criminalizing the mentally compromised. My clients are as brain-injured as victims of Strokes or Alzheimer's Disease.

The Government refuses to recognize Fetal Alcohol Syndrome as the single biggest cause for jail overcrowding and overloaded probation officers, overworked judges and overworked prosecutors.

They are Labelled Anti-Social

I failed to see that if my clients were old, with Alzheimer's Disease, instead of 20 years old, male and with a long Criminal Record, they would be getting many services. Instead they are labeled as "anti-social" and sent to jail.

The First Step

This paper argues for systemic change. This paper hopes to persuade you, the reader, that the first step in preparing for Court is securing an Assessment for Fetal Alcohol Syndrome by doctors trained in assessing Fetal Alcohol Syndrome. In B.C., this is available, at present, only at the Asante Centre in Maple Ridge, which specializes in Fetal Alcohol Syndrome Assessments. Fetal Alcohol Syndrome Assessments are not available anywhere else in British Columbia, although they are readily available in Seattle, Calgary and Edmonton.

I am Now Applying

As a lawyer, I am now applying to the Provincial Court for an Order pursuant to Section 723(3) of the *Criminal Code of Canada* that the British Columbia Government, specifically the Minister of Health or the Attorney General, to pay for the Asante Centre to prepare a Fetal Alcohol Syndrome Assessment.

Everyone Needs to Know

My client is going to jail. Lawyers, police, corrections officials, probation officers, the family, and, most of all, the clients need to know about Fetal Alcohol Syndrome and how Fetal Alcohol Syndrome has affected my client. The B.C. Government refuses to pay for a Fetal Alcohol Syndrome

Assessment. The Legal Services Society also refuses to pay for a Fetal Alcohol Syndrome Assessment. This is wrong. I hope a Judge will order that the Attorney General pay for such a needed procedure. Forensic Psychiatric Services admits that its medical staff have no specialized expertise in the area of Fetal Alcohol Syndrome.

The Process of My Education

The process of my education has been an accelerated and sad learning curve. Unfortunately, my clients suffered because I had to learn the hard way. My clients did not have a proper Fetal Alcohol Syndrome Assessment because I failed to consider it some six years ago.

Will I see these clients again? I am certain of it. It is my hope that a routine assessment for Fetal Alcohol Syndrome is made for each new client who enters the criminal justice system. An assessment done today will cut down on repeat crime, save money for the judicial system, and save years of heartbreak for the families.

New Understanding of FASD in Canadian Prisons

The criminal justice system, especially corrections and prison settings, could attempt intervention efforts rather that isolation and punishment. Health Canada offered an 11 million dollar initiative, to be spent over 3 years, to enhance FASD activities related to public awareness and training, education and capacity development, early identification and diagnosis. This was announced in August 2000. The initiative will be based on existing programming, as well as undertaking new projects.

Health and Social Services Minister Don Roberts announced that the government has amended the Yukon Public Health Act to require all physicians to report a diagnosis of FAS to a central registry. The information is intended to help better target prevention, treatment and support programs. Numbers can be counted but individual privacy protected.

In an unpublished study described by Streissguth (1997), in a Washington State prison it was discovered that the profile of behavioral characteristics of adults with FASD was well known to corrections officers. They were unaware there was a name for the profile. In prisons now, with the heightened awareness, Corrections Canada is looking at new services for FASD individuals. The primary requirements are to be able to identify these individuals in order to offer the correct treatment need and design.

Recommendations from Corrections Services Canada include identifying individuals with FASD, offering correctional programs that will consider the dysfunction of the individual, and if there are sufficient numbers with FAS, they would consider appointing an advocate to help this population. They also suggest that CSC design an FASD manual and implement in-service training in order to educate and raise awareness. There was also the recognition that because of their permanent neurological deficits and many secondary problems, FAS inmates would require extensive planning for their release.

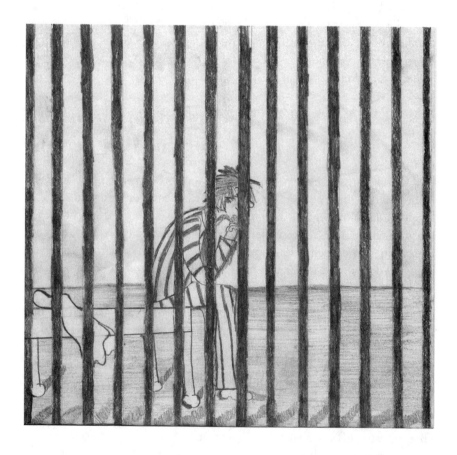

Social Programming: What Works

Harm Reduction: Washington Prevention Model Takes off in Alberta

by Pam van Vugt

The P-CAP (Parent-Child Assistance Project) is a prevention program for decreasing the number of babies born with FASD (Fetal Alcohol Spectrum Disorder) and/or the number of babies born affected by drugs.

The program is based on the Seattle, University of Washington's P-CAP program, which has been running since 1991. P-CAP is a model for intervening with high-risk substance-abusing mothers though the use of paraprofessionals and a home visiting model. The program focuses on high-risk women who have received little or no prenatal care and are not connected to community resources. The principal issues being addressed are drug and alcohol treatment, family planning, child safety and stability, and the prevention of future alcohol- and drug-exposed infants.

The background of mothers enrolled in the P-CAP program is characterized by poverty, upbringing by substance-abusing parents, childhood abuse, abusive adult relationships, trouble with the law, and chaotic and unstable living conditions. As products of this background, they often distrust community service agencies and are disconnected from social networks.

The goals of P-CAP are:

- To assist clients in getting alcohol and drug treatment, staying in recovery, and resolving complex problems that have arisen during the period of their substance abuse.

- To assure that the children of these mothers are in a safe home environment and receive appropriate health care.

- To link mothers to community resources for professional services and education that will help them build and maintain healthy independent family lives.

- To demonstrate to community services providers, strategies for working with women who are often considered hopeless, in order to prevent the future births of affected babies.

Program/Service Components

P-CAP is a home visitation program. The home visitors are paraprofessional advocates who have commonalities with the clients in regards to personal histories and cultural backgrounds. Long term (3 years) relationships are built with at risk moms with a focus on bridging the gap between the clients and appropriate community resources. The essential element of this model is personalized, caring support over a long enough period of time to allow for gradual, enduring changes to occur. The successful implementation of these long term caring relationships is dependent upon the effective use of paraprofessionals. These paraprofessionals, Parents Advocates, serve as positive role models; provide practical in-home assistance; link the clients with professionals in the community; and establish strong communication networks among service providers supporting individual clients. The advocates are responsible for a caseload of 12-15 clients. Concrete methods, including the signing of written agreements, are used to help identify personal goals and the steps necessary to meet those goals. Cultural diversity is reflected in this program and components will be modified accordingly. Advocates do not provide direct services, but coordinate and utilize community health, drug treatment and social services. They are available by pagers. Intensity and frequency of contact can range from daily to twice per month.

P-CAP used two models for its theoretical framework. The two theories are Relational Theory and Harm Reduction Theory. P-CAP uses three approaches or interventions – Model of Change, Motivational Interviewing and Structured Program Activities.

Advocates also follow McMan's Service Delivery Model, which involves:

1. Single point of entry – Program Supervisor coordinates all referrals
2. Commencement
3. Identify and agree on issues/needs
4. Assessment and Intervention
5. Ending the Helping Relationship
6. Evaluating Service Delivery and Outcomes

As P-CAP in Seattle is a research model, information is collected on the women. All women are given an Addiction Severity Index upon entry to and exit from the program. Information is collected bi-annually from all clients. At this point the information is used for statistical analysis only. All analysis is done by number.

Preventing FASD:
The Challenges of Programming
for High Risk Mothers in Alberta

by Mary Berube

As with any program that attempts to influence the lives of clients that have longstanding issues, the First Steps program has run into many challenges and hurdles in the first three years of service.

Finding appropriate housing for our clients has become the single most time consuming issue the mentors encounter when intervening with this population. Not only is acquiring housing very difficult because of the acute shortage of affordable and/or subsidized housing, but when housing is available, the cost of rent far exceeds the monthly rates paid out by SFI. The SFI (welfare) rate does not even cover basic cost of rent, let alone the cost of food and utilities, or transportation and clothing, thus necessitating many trips to the food bank and clothing exchanges. Those women who have been involved in the sex-trade are tempted find an unconventional solution to this shortage – they turn a few tricks with either former customers or the landlord in order to make ends meet. Many landlords are reluctant to rent to these clients, and they have no money for the damage deposit or to hook up their utilities, often due to their past poor performance.

When child protection is considering returning children home to a mother, she runs into difficulty because when she is alone, she is not eligible to have access to subsidized housing or SFI rates for rentals that contain more than one bedroom, and she is not eligible to have her children with her until she has enough bedrooms in her home, so she is caught in a circular argument which she cannot win. Only very skilled advocacy has ever managed to address this strange barrier to normalcy.

When she wants to enter a residential alcohol or drug treatment program, she is in danger of losing her home if SFI does not consent to pay both rent and room and board.

Many of the women have experienced sexual abuse and will require assistance to overcome the effects this has had on their lives. A significant proportion have been involved in prostitution and they are likely suffering from post traumatic stress syndrome as a consequence. This, too, will need to be addressed at some point in their recovery. Many have been prescribed medication for mental health issues and several others would be appropriate for a referral to assess their need for medication. Those women who have criminal records have some rather unpleasant unfinished business to take care of, including doing time.

Another concern we have with regards to our clients revolves around their long-term ability to sustain sobriety. We have managed to enrol many of them in treatment. However, she may lose temporary custody of her children if the program has no room for them, and most do not. Many programs are co-ed and these clients are not able to handle the stress of relating to males in addition to treatment. This may mean they have enormous difficulty staying with the program for the prescribed length of time. Conversely, most programs are not long enough to help the women regain a stable foothold as a fully functioning member of society. Once out of treatment, managing to stay clean and sober over the long run presents them with so many challenges; creating a new pattern of behavior in varied circumstances, creating or re-creating habits that come with a clean lifestyle, learning life skills, finding legitimate means of earning a living, relating to partners and family in new ways, leaving behind those persons in their lives who are not helpful to the process, reclaiming children, addressing their health issues, and including reliable and sensible family planning.

Another issue that we have identified in the course of working with our clients concerns their ability to parent. So many of these women have had very poor beginnings themselves in life with regards to being parented. They come from backgrounds that most of us would characterize as predominantly dysfunctional and have often been in substitute or foster care at least once. They have no good models for parenting and are out of practice because they have frequently not cared for their own children for any significant length of time. While their babies are very young and cute, they seem to be quite attached to them, but as soon as the child begins the arduous process of growing up and challenging the mother, she tends to become quickly discouraged and impatient and/or finds alternate care arrangements for the child. She may also soon have another on the way unless she has been helped to see how unwise this is. Not only does parenting require a very long time commitment, it will require, for many of these women, a

Herculean effort to overcome their own poor beginnings. Any who are parenting alcohol- and drug-affected children, with all of the additional problems that attend that disability, will have the odds stacked against them even higher.

The majority of our clients tend to have rather poor self-esteem because they are disappointed in themselves, others and their lives, and because of the many negative messages they have received about themselves. They have a tendency to blame others for most or all of their mistakes and circumstances and have trouble accepting that they have a part in how their lives have turned out. Our role is to be both supportive and confrontational when needed, in order to address this issue. Long term repair of damaged self-esteem with the antecedents that are present here, will take enormous energy on the part of both mentor and client.

A significant number of these clients have themselves been exposed to alcohol in utero. They demonstrate all of the characteristics that come with this exposure and will require a mentor or helper for life. Three years will not be enough to stem the tide of harm that had been incurred in these women's lives. Additionally, they will need a diagnosis and assessment in order for us to help them effectively.

In spite of all of the previously mentioned concerns, the women demonstrate several positive characteristics that have been encouraging.

- They are tenacious. They have not given up hope for a better life.
- Many have been very committed to having involvement with a mentor and the program and believe this to be a good investment of their time and energy.
- They are getting to know their children and want to be reunited with them and become reconnected with their families.
- They have increased their level of sobriety during the target pregnancy when they have the services of a mentor.
- Their housing situations have improved.
- They have expressed interest in, and have done something positive about their former lack of reproductive health. They are interested in becoming free of sexually transmitted diseases. They want to have healthy babies, and they are prepared to postpone pregnancy in order to achieve this.
- They want to work towards legal and stable employment.

Aim of Program

To replicate and adapt, where appropriate, the "Birth to Three/PCAP" Program model (as designed by the University of Washington in Seattle) within the City of Edmonton.

To reduce the number of births that are pre-natally exposed to alcohol and/or drugs, and to prevent the recurrence of births amongst the most high-risk women in Edmonton.

To create learning opportunities for other agencies that wish to replicate this program through training and through sharing information and data.

Target Population

Women at high risk of having a pregnancy concurrent with alcohol and/or drug exposure, who are currently pregnant or up to 6 months post-partum and who are not effectively linked to existing services.

Women who themselves have FASD and are at risk of simultaneously using drugs/alcohol and being pregnant, and who are not effectively linked to existing services.

Women who have a previous child diagnosed with FASD, are currently pregnant, and at risk of relapsing with regards to drug/alcohol use and are not effectively linked to services in Edmonton.

Referral Sources

- Neo-natal intensive care unit staff
- Addictions counselors
- Self-referrals/referrals from acquaintances
- Community health nurses
- Justice
- Child protection workers
- Staff at local birthing units
- Physicians
- Community agencies
- Home visitation projects
- Therapists

Goals

We have two main program goals:

1. Reduce the number of births the client has that are alcohol/drug exposed.

2. Address the well-being of the target child.

Technically, by not drinking or abusing drugs during pregnancy, FASD is entirely preventable. However, this is not easy for those women who have little or no self-esteem, have no formal education, live in poverty and abuse, and have no support system to turn to for help. These women may not be aware of the dire consequences of chemical dependency during pregnancy or may not have the skills and confidence necessary to change their lives. It is only natural that these women with extremely complicated and dysfunctional lives feel hopeless.

The First Step Fetal Alcohol Syndrome/Effects Pilot Prevention Program was begun in 1999 and provides one-to-one educational, social and outreach supports services to women at risk of giving birth to a child with FASD. This group is comprised of females between the ages of 18 and 36 who have been identified by various social, health and child welfare agencies, hospitals and community professionals (i.e., social workers, medical doctors, school principals, lawyers, etc.). The program was designed to assist women at highest risk of giving birth to a child with Fetal Alcohol Syndrome, who are either pregnant or have recently given birth. Women are matched with a mentor who will work one-on-one with them for three years to assist them in ordering their lives and establishing a healthy, positive lifestyle for themselves and their children.

For perhaps the first time in the lives of the women, they have a consistent support person to whom they can turn for help, who is always there for them and who will not judge them for the choices they have made. While the mentor assists with developing life skills, they also provide the women with someone to count on and to reach out to in times of need – someone they can trust and with whom they feel comfortable; someone who understands that relapse is normal.

Women who participate in the program receive practical and reliable help in many domains – drug/alcohol rehabilitation; parenting; freedom from abuse; self-esteem; and understanding the "system" (i.e., Child Welfare, Supports for Independence, and the law and its language.) Their mentor will be with them at Child Welfare, probation officer and lawyer meetings; when they enter drug/alcohol rehabilitation centres; at maintenance enforcement hearings; during court appearances and medical appointments and meetings with landlords.

Prenatal substance abuse carries a significant price tag in direct and indirect costs to both mother and child. It also has overwhelming and deleterious ramifications for the inividuals affected and the community at large. It is estimated that in the Province of Alberta, 5%-15% of the population has FAS/E. Knowledgeable medical personnel and social work practitioners have suggested that 35%-45% of the nearly 12 000 children in care of the department of Child Welfare in the Province of Alberta suffer from FASD. Clinical experience in the province suggests that nearly 30%-40% of young offenders and adult prison inmates suffer from the debilitating effects of FASD.

FASD is an irrevocable life sentence – for the child who has an altered developmental trajectory from birth, and a life sentence of social, financial, judicial, educational and medical costs and services that must then be provided by the government or community in order to care for this person from birth through adulthood. The only way to address these costs is through prevention.

Expected Outcomes

We evaluate the Program at multiple levels. The five domains on which we regularly report to the funders are:

- Alcohol/Drug Treatment
- Abstinence from Alcohol/Drugs
- Reproductive Health
- Well-being of Target Child
- Effective Connections to Services

The outcomes that we plan to survey at the end of the 3 years include:

Participants completing the program have achieved increased physical, emotional, mental, spiritual, social and economic well-being.

Participant has experienced a long-term, trusting relationship with Mentor, and has begun to establish other such relationships.

Participant is effectively connected with resources that provide appropriate concrete support.

Participant is able to assess current situation and to identify and communicate her own strengths, resources, needs and aspirations independently, or has the support to do so.

Participants are able to explain their (dis)ability to others.

Participants have attained personal goals established throughout the program.

Participants know how to set goals and to plan for their achievement either independently or with support.

Program Components

Providing intensive home visiting, support and advocacy to women at risk of having a child with FASD with the explicit aim of building self-advocacy skills and positive mutual support networks.

Identification of service barriers through working with the client and her family.

Building supports and removing barriers encountered by individuals impacted by FASD through advocacy, case conferencing, meaningful participation in the life of the community and modeling holistic strengths-oriented services.

Raising awareness of FASD and related issues through individual contacts and wherever it is appropriate, and through presentations developed in conjunction with training co-ordinator and/or community team.

Participating in evaluation activities that support evidenced-based, reflective practice and enhance the project's ability to achieve its expected outcomes.

Case loads range from 12-15 clients to each mentor. Intake worker will handle up to 30 clients.

Dimensions of Practice

We have adopted the critical elements of the Birth to 3 Model as follows:

Members never give up on participants; participants are never asked to leave the program.

Participants define and evaluate personal goals every 6 months, which mentors co-ordinate with program goals.

Developing a network of relationships with everyone involved in a participant's life.

The program provides advocacy for other family/social network members as needed.

Connecting a participant's service providers with each other to create an effective plan.

The program does not provide direct services, but links the participant with the best available community service and identifies and actively resolves existing service barriers.

Assisting in developing individualized case plans with mother, the justice system, and child welfare, and any other service providers when Child Protection is involved.

The program continues to provide a mentor for both mother and target child, regardless of custody issues.

Mandatory individual weekly supervision of each mentor by the clinical supervisor, and mandatory weekly group staffing sessions. These factors enables the entire team to learn from the progress of each other's clients, provides for ongoing training, and allows visiting community professionals an opportunity to experience the program.

Ongoing program evaluation generates information on a regular basis that is used by the program to enhance the work of advocacy.

Theoretical Approaches

Motivational Interviewing/Stages of Change

Strengths Orientation/Solution Focused

Relational Theory, Mentoring Model *

*Five key principles of coaching

1. Relationship – trust and respect
2. Pragmatism – replaces theory
3. Learning – reciprocal for both parties
4. Adapting to the needs of the client
5. Techniques

Workers' Qualifications

Minimum 2 years post secondary in Social Work or related area.

5 years minimum experience in working with high-risk populations.

Support Provided to Workers

Intense pre-service training* (80-100 hours approx)

Minimum 40-60 hours per year of subsequent training

Weekly clinical supervision.

Weekly group case conferencing.

Supervision as needed.

Yearly performance evaluations.

Feedback from client evaluation results to provide guidance and good news.

Provide competitive salary and benefits to maintain worker well-being and prevent staff turnover.

Evaluation Results

So far, we are very gratified by the results of our interventions.

There have been no new ETOH/drug impacted births to program participants in the first 2 years. Previously, these clients were having drug/ETOH-exposed babies every 12 to 18 months.

The women report a high rate of satisfaction with the mentors and with the program.

No staff turn over.

Example of Client Success

"Alice" came to First Steps two days after the birth of her baby. When we met her, she was desperate and gratefully accepted help. Her baby's toxicology tests showed traces of cocaine. Alice admitted to using drugs and alcohol throughout the pregnancy. Alice was terrified that Child Welfare was going to take her beautiful new baby because previously, her two other children had been apprehended. Child Welfare did, in fact, plan to apprehend the baby, but agreed to wait because she had a First Steps program mentor involved to support her through rough times.

In less than three months, there has been a dramatic change in the quality of Alice's life. Each success furthers brightens her spirits and raises her self-esteem. With her mentor's guidance and support, Alice has achieved the following:

-   She has remained free of alcohol and drugs, and has followed through with regular substance abuse counselling;

- She has followed through on all requirements of her probation officer, regular visits have been replaced by monthly phone calls;
- A Permanent Guardianship Order for her two other children was changed to a Temporary Guardianship Order because mom was making signs of progress;
- She is nursing her baby, and it is healthy, happy and strong;
- Alice insisted that her common-law partner leave unless he, too could stay clean and sober. After leaving for a couple of weeks, he came back willing to cooperate. He is now taking classes in preparation for a work training program that begins next month.
- Alice has gone from one supervised visit every two weeks with the children in foster care, to one unsupervised overnight visit each week;
- She has been given a stay on proceedings on all upcoming court appearances for numerous criminal offences because she has proven to the court that she is making considerable changes in her life.
- After learning about family planning, she has made an appointment to have her tubes tied to prevent further pregnancy.

Step by Step Program

Agency

Catholic Social Services

Aim of Program

- Reduce the breakdown of appropriate parent-child relationships, resulting in apprehension and placement of children in the care of Alberta Child and Family Services.
- Using Individualized Service Plans, each person living with FASD and their families will design specific goals for increased independence and success in the community.
- Prevent the development of secondary disabilities in the lives of both the parent and the children.

Target Population

Women who themselves have FASD and are actively parenting children who are or are not affected by FASD, and who are not effectively linked to existing services.

Referral Sources

- Addictions counselors
- Self-referrals/referrals from acquaintances
- Community health nurses
- Justice
- Child protection workers
- Physicians
- Community agencies
- Home visitation projects
- Therapists

Goals

We have three main program goals:

1. Reduce the breakdown of appropriate parent-child relationships, resulting in apprehension and placement of children in the care of Alberta Child and Family Services.
2. Strengthen parenting and life skills essential to raising successful children.
3. Increase the mother's independence and success in the community.

Additionally, each participant in the program is involved in setting her own goals in the Individualized Service Plan and these are evaluated every six months for the bi-annual assessment, or as necessary to keep client and mentor on track.

Expected Outcomes

We evaluate the Program at multiple levels. The domains on which we regularly report to the funders are:

- Alcohol/Drug Treatment
- Parenting skills
- Coping skills

- Life skills
- Work/Education skills
- Recreational Involvement
- Supportive family involvement
- Effective Connections to Services

The outcomes that we plan to survey at the end of the 3 years include:

- Participants completing the program have achieved increased physical, emotional, mental, spiritual, social and economic well-being.
- Participant has experienced a long-term, trusting relationship with Mentor, and has begun to establish other such relationships.
- Participant is effectively connected with resources that provide appropriate concrete support.
- Participant is able to assess current situation and to identify and communicate her own strengths, resources, needs and aspirations independently, or has the support to do so.
- Participants are able to explain their (dis)ability to others.
- Participants have attained personal goals established throughout the program.
- Participants know how to set goals and to plan for their achievement either independently or with support.

Program Components

This will involve intensive home visiting, support and advocacy to women with FASD who are raising children with the explicit aim of building up those skills and networks essential to raising successful children.

Identification of service barriers through working with the client and her family.

Building supports and removing barriers encountered by individuals impacted by FASD through advocacy, case conferencing, meaningful participation in the life of the community and modeling holistic strengths-oriented services.

Raising awareness of FASD and related issues through individual contacts and wherever it is appropriate, and through presentations developed in conjunction with training co-ordinator and/or community team.

Participating in evaluation activities that support evidenced-based, reflective practice and enhance the project's ability to achieve its expected outcomes.

Case loads range from 6-8 clients for each mentor.

Dimensions of Practice

We have adopted the critical elements of the First Steps Model as follows:

Members never give up on participants; participants are never asked to leave the program.

Participants and mentors define and evaluate personal goals every 6 months as laid out in the Individualized Service Plan.

Developing a network of relationships with everyone involved in a participant's life.

The program provides advocacy for other family/social network members as needed.

Connecting a participant's service providers with each other to create an effective plan.

The program does not provide direct services, but links the participant with the best available community service and identifies and actively resolves existing service barriers.

Assisting in developing individualized case plans with mother, the justice system, and child welfare, and any other service providers.

Mandatory individual weekly supervision of each mentor by the clinical supervisor, and mandatory weekly group staffing sessions. These factors enable the entire team to learn from the progress of each other's clients, provides for ongoing training, and allows visiting community professionals an opportunity to experience the program.

Ongoing program evaluation generates information on a regular basis that is used by the program to enhance the work of advocacy.

An Experience in Advocacy

A couple of weeks ago, Debbie and I attempted to get an extenuation on her "Fine Option" program. Debbie had had a year to complete the necessary hours to pay off her fines, but she had failed to do so. We went to the courthouses where she applied for an extenuation. Debbie was told that her application would be given to a judge and she would be called with the results within two days. Unfortunately, her application for extenuation was denied. She only had until October 31/00 to rectify the matter as this was the deadline for completion of her "Fine Options" agreement. On Thursday, October 26/00, I helped Debbie write a letter of appeal and I wrote a letter advocating on her behalf. Debbie was to take this to the courthouse on Friday, October 27/00. I offered to drive her there, but she assured me that she had a ride and would do this herself.

Normally, Debbie would call immediately to tell me how things went. I did not receive a call on Friday, nor did she answer my calls. This "silence" continued through Monday, October 30, and Tuesday October 31. I was really beginning to worry about Debbie so, even though she wasn't answering my calls, I went to her house. The house looked very suspicious – there were blankets over all the windows. I knocked and knocked, yelling, "Debbie, I know you are in there!" Finally, Debbie came to the door. She looked like she had been crying and was extremely unkempt in her appearance. After some encouragement, she finally told me what was wrong. She had "crashed" on the previous Friday, and had been on a bender right through to Monday night. She was feeling ashamed and angry with herself. In addition, she had not gone to the courthouse the previous Friday to appeal the court's denial of an extenuation to her "Fine Options." Now, it was November 1/00 and the deadline had passed – there would be a warrant out for her arrest. In her depression, she was assuming the worst. She was sure that she would go to jail and Child Welfare would take her baby away. At that moment, I wasn't sure what I was going to do, but I encouraged her to get cleaned up and dressed. I knew that the problem wouldn't simply go away simply by hiding behind blanketed windows. We got the baby dressed too, and off we went. Debbie asked, "Where are we going?" I answered, "To court – what have we go to lose?" We finally arrived at court. We went to a counter marked "Criminal Division" where I explained the circumstances and asked what steps we could take to rectify the problem. The court clerk was quite abrupt indicating repeatedly that the deadline had passed and there would be a warrant. I held my ground saying, "There must be something we can do." The clerk said that the only way would be to appear in person before a judge, but she did not recommend that as Debbie could be arrested immediately. I said, "That is a chance we'll take!" I asked in which courtroom I could find a judge presently sitting. The clerk said, "Now?" I replied, "Now." We were directed to Courtroom Number 268. Debbie was scared and anxious, but I said that even if she is arrested, it is better to get it over with than to live in fear. Besides, I would be there to help make the necessary arrangements for the baby. Finally, Debbie agreed and off we went.

Debbie could not come into the courtroom because infants are not allowed inside. She promised to wait outside the courtroom while I went in to try and figure out how we might get before the judge. I went in and sat down, watching the various cases. I decided to write out our problem in the form of a letter and take it up to the prosecuting attorney at the front of the courtroom. This I did and quietly went and sat down again. Soon the attorney looked my way and nodded, "Okay." I immediately went outside the courtroom and told Debbie that she would be soon called, at which point I would come out and get her. I encouraged her to, in the meantime, find a court worker to look after the baby for a few minutes while she went into the courtroom. Very soon, the two of us were before the judge. I explained the situation to the judge indicating that even though Debbie had a full year to work off her fines, there were extenuating circumstances that prevented this from happening – like a pregnancy with complications and the birth of her baby. I further indicated that Debbie is now ready to go work, a work placement has been arranged at Abbotsfield Mall, and appropriate child care has been found. Then, I submitted Debbie's letter and my letter of advocacy. Soon the judge said, "Well, this isn't normally a court of appeal for the "Fine Option" program, but I am willing to grant you six months if you feel this would be enough. I appreciate this kind of effort of your part, Debbie, and I admire your advocacy, Ms. –. As these letters aren't submitted as official evidence, normally I would give them back. However, I would very much like to keep them if I may. You two have made my day, I wish you the very best…and, how is your baby, Debbie?"

Debbie learned a lot that day. In tears of happiness she said, "I'll never run away from a problem again….and you really can get respect when you try to do what is right."

Coaching Families Program

Agency

Catholic Social Services

Aim of Program

To improve the well being and stability of individuals with FASD and their families.

The program will work to enhance protective factors with regards to decreasing the incidence of secondary disabilities of FASD and decrease risk behaviors through:

- providing crisis intervention
- support to appropriately adjust expectations and environments of individuals with FASD
- effectively linking participants to appropriate ongoing support

Target Population

Caregivers of children aged 0-18 who have been diagnosed with FASD or who demonstrate strong behavioral and learning indicators of prenatal exposure to alcohol are eligible for program support.

Referral Sources

- Self
- Services to Children with Disabilities
- Community
- Child Protection Workers

Expected Outcomes

Expected outcomes of our program include:

- Demonstrated improvement in knowledge of FASD and increased capacity to address issues related to FASD among caregivers, other family members and service providers
- Improved access to diagnosis and family support services across the region
- A greater capacity of identifying FASD within families and preventing subsequent births of children prenatally exposed to alcohol
- Increased capacity in other professionals to screen for FASD
- Decreased rates of secondary disabilities in affected individuals
- Decrease rates of parent burnout and placement disruption

End of Program outcomes surveyed on completion of services include:

- Participants having a better understanding of FASD and demonstrate appropriate coping skills

- Participants effectively connected with community resources that enhance and sustain their coping skills
- Participants are able to advocate for themselves and their child(ren)
- Participants are attending a support group (formed by the program)

Goals

- To ensure the families/caregivers are well connected to the community and to each other with a variety of supports
- Increase the understanding and knowledge of FASD among families, caregivers and other community supports
- Improve the well being and stability of individuals with FASD and their families by enhancing protective factors and decreasing risk factors
- Provide families with strategies and tools to decrease the risk of secondary disabilities
- Build on family strengths
- Ensure the children are in a safe and stable environment

Program Components

- Provide In-Home Support for a period of 3-6 months to enhance protective factors and to prevent secondary disabilities. Services provided are on a basis similar to the mentorship model used in the existing First Steps Program. In this model, services are provided in a one-on-one fashion with an emphasis on direct helping.
- Needs and Strengths Assessment of the affected child(ren) and the family/caregiver
- Determine understanding and implications of the FASD diagnosis, including possible issues of grief and loss, and the prevention of parent burnout, and reduction of placement disruption
- Educating and training the family and community service providers about FASD issues
- Teach, assist and support the family/caregiver in constructing environments best suited for themselves and their affected child(ren)
    a) Work with Community to raise awareness and understanding of special services required and of effective interventions where FASD is a factor. As well, the program will assist and teach others to adapt programs and services to the needs of the family, including

adding capacity to existing multi-disciplinary teams to identify possible FASD, to effectively intervene where FASD may be a factor, and to refer for diagnosis and assessment.

- Consultation and assistance with Case Management Plans in a multi-disciplinary team setting, and with other Service Providers, often collaborating with Child Protection Services. Also, consultation and needs assessment for other Service Providers

- Consultation and collaboration with Services to Children with Disabilities for the provision of respite to prevent secondary disabilities caused through placement disruption

- Referral and Advocacy: training the family to effectively acquire services, deal with crises and assist in case management plans. The advocacy on behalf of families will also be to teach members of the professional community and the general public to screen for FASD

  b) Offer sustained support to families once the mentor has phased out of the helping process

- Provide community resources, including referrals to the First Steps program when appropriate to prevent any new children being born with FASD

- Link families to community supports and with schools in order to establish parallel structures, from home, for the children

- Encourage families to attend a support group

- Families are encouraged to receive telephone support from the mentors, during the next few months, and can re-enter the program if required

Dimensions of Practice

1. The service provided by the program is voluntary

2. The service provided by the program is free to clients

3. The program engages the family/caregiver in a process which will help them adjust to life with FASD

4. The program ensures families/caregivers are effectively linked to resources and to others

5. Clients can return to the program, and are welcome to contact the program at any time after

6. Goals are set by and with clients for expectations of our involvement

7. The program provides advocacy for other family/social network members as needed

8. Connect the service providers to each other in order to create an effective plan for the family

9. Assist in developing case plans with the family and other service providers

10. Weekly supervision by the clinical supervisor is mandatory

11. Ongoing program evaluation generates information on a regular basis that is used by the program to enhance the work of advocacy

12. Case loads range from 9 to 14 (there are presently 4 mentors)

13. Interventionists will work with the Glenrose Diagnostic Team when completing assessments.

Evaluation

We evaluate the Program using pre and post measures including stress evaluation, and needs assessment of clients. The program also measures the achievement of Individual Service Plan goals by each family as recorded and measured on the Hull Outcome Monitoring and Evaluation System (HOMES)

- Participants have become involved in our support group
- Participants have expressed relief and high satisfaction to have the support of our program
- Participants have expressed effective connection to community services
- No staff turn over

Sun Dance

by Diane Wrubleski

Spirit healer
One with our forefathers
Remind me that I only have this day
Yesterday is past and tomorrow never comes
Help me to achieve my goals
Before the day is done
Impart to me the wisdom of my ancestors
Heal me with the spirit of the Mother Earth
Strengthen me to meet the storm
To face adversity
And find courage to walk through hardship
Instill in me the patience of the buffalo
The strength of the bear
The swiftness of the antelope
The ability to reach the eagle's heights
Nurture me in the circle of my sisters and brothers
Bestow on me a kinder, gentler soul
That counts my neighbour in my clan
Where every life has value equal to my own
Dance in the sun with me to celebrate new life
Rejoice in new beginnings
To see the good in every circumstance
The beauty in a blizzard
And the promise in a rainbow
Remind me to give much more than I receive
And reap the blessings of that honor
Help me to laugh to cleanse my heart
And free my soul
Help me to learn from my mistakes
And gain a higher understanding
To accept myself and my beginnings
Uplift me on your wings
And watch me dance
Spirit Healer

Family Stories

Supporting Caregivers Through the Difficulties

As we actively listened to parents and full time care providers, we heard a similar story over and over. It went like this: *When we began to foster or accept this child into our world, we had no idea what the future looked like for our family. We saw problems, searched for answers, often the birth mom's pregnancy was unknown and we needed answers, but we received very little that seemed to fit or help us go in the right direction. It was sink or swim, it was overwhelming, exhausting and we truly needed to be believed, not be disciplined or offered a parenting class!*

Parents need to be listened to and supported. They need to be given the acknowledgment of their expertise in raising their children.

Parenting in many regards is a public endeavor. To assume the role of parent to a child, is to accept a certain amount of public praise or scrutiny regarding their child and their ability as parents. Just as an author is judged by the quality of their metaphors and the potency of their language, the quality of a parent is largely judged by how well their children adjust and function in the world beyond their doorstep. If their children are successful, parents share their children's sense of pride and accomplishment. But if children become entangled in trouble, parents shoulder much of the blame. In relation to FASD, the gradient by which we judge the success of a parent must be drastically adjusted.

My child is charming and excellent at not telling the truth to teachers, social workers or community members. As a result they took the child's word over mine; this amazed me given that I am a good care provider and I know and tried to explain that manipulation and dishonesty are a part of the coping mechanisms for individuals with FASD. I was insulted they believed the child over me.

— Louise

It must be understood that many traditional methods of parenting are simply not sufficient with children with FASD. For example if you caught your ten-year-old daughter stealing money from your purse, the accepted course of action would be to discipline her, first by explaining why you were angry, why what she was doing was wrong and why she should not repeat her behavior. Chances are if the consequences were severe enough, she would not repeat the same action. If this child had FASD, you could discipline her more than a dozen times, you could talk until you are blue in the face, but the behavior would continue. Though public and professional awareness about FASD has been steadily increasing over the three decades following its discovery, few individuals in the professional community have a sincere understanding of the daily challenges involved in raising a child with FASD. This knowledge only comes with first hand experience. In raising a child with FASD, parents and their community support network must develop new methods by which to measure their child's and their own success.

> *I had to go away on business for a few weeks. I left my child, who was ten at the time, in the care of a friend. Prior to my departure we went over the rules and reviewed the challenges she might face due to the fact that my child had FAE. The baby sitter was a mother herself and very conscientious. Upon my return the babysitter shared this comment: "I know you informed me of what to expect with Pat but I was not prepared for what I experienced; the lack of follow through, the forgetfulness, the mistakes, the lack of common sense. Experiencing is believing. I have a new respect for your work and a new understanding of FAE."*
>
> *– Samantha*

It is so important to listen to the caregivers who provide full-time care. FASD is not an easy diagnosis, especially the invisible FAE. Many parents have asked this question: "Why don't professionals listen when we speak? They interact with our children for short periods of time and then make judgements about our parenting skills. We live with these children ever day, we witness the big picture. We know that something is very wrong with this child regardless of what the teachers, doctors and social workers say."

Casual interviews in a relaxed environment with the promise of anonymity allowed for candid responses about living with FASD. We spoke with three adoptive mothers who discovered the FASD diagnosis later in the adoption. Before reaching the FAS diagnosis, they collectively saw many professionals, often each have a different theory regarding the learning problems and behaviors.

All three women adopted the children as babies, all three had a professional background, one a pediatric nurse, one a program evaluator and the third a social worker. All women are middle class and have exceptional social networking ability. Their backgrounds did not prove as helpful as one might think, when seeking help they were often treated as if they were being difficult or even overbearing regarding their children. One mother was told that perhaps she should take a parenting course. She was taken aback, as she had raised three biological children without consequence and was a nurse specializing in children's care. She felt blamed, not supported and she was amazed at the variety of responses to the situation, leaving her feeling betrayed. There is one glaring truth that seems to be overlooked or minimized in importance; this is the voice of the full-time caregiver. They have valuable information and observations that can be used to assist in understanding this disability. In a *Globe and Mail* article published in 2003, journalist Margaret Philippe made an excellent point regarding the power of advocacy of the middle class. They bring to the FASD struggle great new promise with their skills and ability to access resources and fight for change, there is new wind in the sails again.

For the benefit of society, we must listen to these parents in order to prevent their children from becoming involved in the criminal justice system. We must not judge them but rather offer our support, especially when their children get in trouble with the law. It is sad to report how many foster parents burn out due to fact that they lack an enriched support system. As the African proverb says, it takes a village to raise a child, and with FASD the child requires an attentive and skilled team of professionals and community members dedicated to change. We have heard of three adoptive parents who have committed suicide. That is three too many. Research in both Canada and the US indicates that only 10% of the children with FASD are being raised by their birth mothers. So many times I have seen and heard the frustration of foster parents who do not understand the child's behavior. The foster system must be fair and open minded and assure these home placements every opportunity to succeed by offering high end support.

Joining Forces

Joining Forces is a non-profit society formed by parents to enhance the lives of individuals affected by fetal alcohol and those who care for them. Through family support, promoting public awareness and education, and by encouraging scientific research, Joining Forces works to ensure that those individuals affected by fetal alcohol will reach their inherent potential.

Our Goal

To enhance the well-being of individuals and families affected by fetal alcohol.

Objectives

To maintain a support group for individuals affected by pre-natal exposure to alcohol, their families and caregivers.

To provide advocacy for individuals and caregivers dealing with issues concerning Fetal Alcohol Syndrome and Alcohol Related Neuro-development Disorders

To provide information to the public in the prevention of Fetal Alcohol Syndrome and Alcohol Related Neuro-development Disorders.

To be a community resource for information about Fetal Alcohol Syndrome and Alcohol Related Neuro-development Disorders.

To foster educational opportunities for individuals within the fields of education, justice, medicine, mental health and social systems so that they may more easily recognize individuals affected by Fetal Alcohol Syndrome and Alcohol Related Neuro-development Disorders and thereby provide appropriate assessments, treatments, educational programs, interventions and support services.

What is the FASD Parent Mentorship Project?

The FASD Parent Mentorship Project provides Parent Mentors who offer in-home parent-to-parent support to families affected by Fetal Alcohol Spectrum Disorder (FASD)* for parents of children from ages 0 to 30 years.

In addition, the Mentorship Project offers a Parent/Caregiver Support Group as well as learning opportunities for the family and the community regarding FASD services, resources and initiatives. The FASD Parent Mentorship Project is an initiative of the Region 4 FAS Steering Committee. It is funded by the Alberta Partnership on FAS and administered by Joining Forces – Fetal Alcohol Society.

A Parent Mentor is a parent or long-time caregiver of a child affected by FASD. They have been chosen for their knowledge of FASD, their personal experience in dealing with FASD, their compassion and their aptitude for peer mentorship. A Parent Mentor works with the parents to provide emotional support, validation and encouragement in parenting a child with FASD. A Parent Mentor, where applicable, works with the parents in collaboration with a Family Advocate.

The FASD Family Advocacy Project provides Family Advocates who work with the family and in each family's community to help consolidate community professionals connected with the family into an FASD-informed team. The FASD Family Advocacy Project is also an initiative of the Region 4 FAS Steering Committee. It is funded by the Alberta Partnership on FAS and administered by Renfrew Educational Services for ages 0 to 5 yrs, Hull Child and Family Services for ages 6 to 15 yrs and the Community Services Centre for ages 16 to 30 yrs.

What is a Family Advocate?

A Family Advocate is a professional who has training in a field related to human services.

A Family Advocate promotes long-term, integrated family support plans and, where applicable, works with the family in collaboration with a Parent Mentor.

What Kind of Support Does the Parent Mentor Provide?

Most importantly, the parent mentor will provide you with peer emotional support and validation with respect to the experience of living with FASD. They will encourage you to develop independence and confidence in your ability by helping you obtain information and develop understanding about parenting a child with FASD. They will encourage you in dealing with issues relating to FASD in both your home and in the community. They will encourage you in learning and developing effective daily living strategies. They will encourage you in building a support network specific to your family needs. They will work in collaboration with the Family Advocate and other service providers that may be involved with your family. They will support the cultural diversity of your family.

How Will You Know the Project is Successful?

A Project Director will contact you within a few weeks of being assigned a Parent Mentor. They will ask you a short series of questions relating to the stability of your family, your confidence in your parenting ability, your knowledge of FASD and FASD related resources and your relationship with the Parent Mentor. From then on you will be contacted once per quarter to assess your current situation and your progress to date.

Who Else Besides the Parent Mentor Will Be Working with My Family?

The Parent Mentor assigned to your family will be the primary person working with you, however they will work in collaboration with a Family Advocate if both have been assigned to your family. When working in collaboration with a Family Advocate, the Parent Mentor will share information about you with the Family Advocate to ensure they are providing a consistent plan for your family. The Parent Mentor will share information about their clients on a weekly basis with other members of the Mentorship team and a professional providing clinical consultation to the FASD Parent Mentorship Project. At times you may want the Parent Mentor to offer encouragement in a meeting or have a telephone conversation with other service providers or school personnel. This will be done based on the availability of the Parent Mentor and only if authorized by you in writing. There may be times when the Parent Mentor will not be available due to illness, personal emergencies, holidays, etc. In this situation another Parent Mentor or a Project Director may work with you instead.

An Interview with the Founders

Why was Joining Forces formed?

The formation of Joining Forces was in many ways a response to the frustration that we felt as the caregivers of children with FASD. We wanted to have a voice with which we could establish credibility within the community. As parents of children with FASD, many of us had a lot of wounds, either open wounds or the scars from dealing with professionals. This program itself is based on the groundbreaking concept that we want the parents to be the experts in raising their children.

We had a social worker who did not believe in the existence of FASD. She was convinced that the reason why my children were misbehaving was because my husband and I were bad parents. She was so adamant about helping and protecting our children that she completely ignored her responsibility to support us as parents. For me, this took a huge a chunk out of my self esteem, I had convinced myself that I was a bad parent. So the Joining Forces support group came into being at a really appropriate time, a time when I really needed to be listened to. It was so refreshing to hear from parents who were telling the same stories and were having the same frustrations. Now the credibility I have with social services is outstanding, it is nice to finally receive that validation from them.

Do you think that parents feel as if they are blamed for their children's behavior?

Yes, most of these parents have been bashed by the community, their families, their neighbors, everyone in their life has some degree of criticism about their child's behavior and their ability as parents. Sometimes mothers don't even have credibility with their husbands. As a lot the time their husbands can't understand why their children don't respond to discipline.

"Meeting the needs of FASD can be frustrating and complex if you do not understand the disability." — *Lauren*

It is difficult when almost everything that you ever say about your child is negative. Sometimes it is very hard to focus on the positive, people who are not in the same situation don't understand and often make a suggestion like "maybe you need to take a parenting course." That is not what we need, almost 90% of the participants in our program have taken numerous parenting courses.

What most of these parents need is a place where they feel safe and validated, where they can say that they want to kill their kids and no one is going to criticize them because we have all been there before. They don't necessarily need counseling, they need a place where they can get ideas, a place where they can go to be heard and supported.

Creative Parenting...is very much a part of being a parent to FASD children. We had crazy rules in our house — at least other people would have thought them crazy, but for us it became survival.

Do you think that foster parents and adoptive parents should be warned about all of the hurdles that are part of raising a child with FASD?

The truth is that it is very difficult to make someone really understand the effects that raising a child FASD has on a family. It is really hard to comprehend something that affects you every minute of every single hour of every single day. It is constant and all encompassing. Adoptive/foster parents need to know that this is an ongoing process that will not go away or necessarily get better. It takes a huge amount of energy and resources, it is a 24-hour-a-day, lifetime occupation.

When you read all the information on a government website, the facts that are posted do not address all the potential negative outcomes that may occur when raising a child with FASD. It may be fine and dandy to white wash the situation but at what point are you going to tell these adoptive parents that they could be adopting a child that could be a lifetime behavioral management problem? When is that going to happen? Not addressing the situation in its totality is not fair to the child or to the parent. If you bought a car that didn't have a starter and the salesperson did not tell you, you would be really angry. It is the same thing if you are adopting a child, you have the right to know exactly what you are getting into.

It is imperative that there be a full disclosure of a child's history, both medical and family, when placing a child into a foster or adoptive home. We had no idea or even a hint that there was an FASD diagnosis when our child was placed with us. It took seven years before we figured the situation out. — *Malika*

What changes have you witnessed in the community's understanding of FASD?

I remember four years ago, as parents you were look down upon, you were considered "just a parent." You were not a professional, so you didn't have a voice or say. This has changed. Now people are coming to us for advice on how to parent a child with FASD, we have finally received some recognition.

"Just because a person has a Ph.D. does not mean that they know what is best for my child."

We are not sure if the numbers of children born with FASD are going down, but there are many changes that are taking place in the way that we view alcohol and pregnancy. There are many initiatives that are seeking to educate the public. We hope that once this information blankets the people and once the government truly gets on board with a firm understanding of the dynamics of FASD, we are optimistic that the situation for these children and their parents will continue to improve. There is still work to be done, but the future looks brighter.

The Importance of Diagnosis

"We finally knew what we were dealing with!" — *Simone*

It is essential for the caregivers to receive an accurate diagnosis. The families are often flooded with relief to know that there is a name for what they are coping with and most importantly, that hope is available for the future. When parents of FASD reach out to service providers, doctors, teachers, social workers, they are looking for answers, asking to be listened to carefully and taken seriously, they are looking for help. The solutions to working with the FASD individual are not simple. In fact there is nothing simple about this disability due to the many different variables at play; it crosses socio-economic boundaries, it can impact any woman of childbearing age who might have been drinking in pregnancy. The diagnosis is just a guideline, a starting point to working with a life-long disability.

"It is much easier to receive help, understanding and offer guidance if you know what you are dealing with, it eased our frustration."

— Jacqueline

It makes a world of difference to have a diagnosis, even if it is considered by some to be a label. Labeling a child with the name of a disorder has recently received a fair share of controversy. If we reframe the situation to addressing an individual living with a disorder, it is no longer a judgmental label but rather a diagnosis and guidelines for help. Recognizing a diagnosis is crucial to understanding a child's capabilities and weaknesses. FASD does not describe a child, it describes an aspect of child's life that must be respected and acknowledged. The disorder may be part of who they are, but it is not all that they have to offer. FASD does not affect each child in a uniform fashion, it means that in many ways a person with FASD may interact with the world in a different way because they process information in a different way than the rest of the population. That does not mean that persons with FASD are all the same, there is vast diversity within the sphere of the diagnosis. Each individual is unique, with their own personalities, talents and passions.

The best example for me of the benefit of diagnosis is the impact this had on my son's life. When he had "normal" expectations because he is a very handsome, charming boy, he suffered and was misunderstood, frustrated and felt isolated, where as knowing about his FAE has given him answers, help and hope. I asked him about how he felt about his diagnosis, he said, "Mom, of course I wanted to know, cause I always knew I was different and sad about not doing well in school, knowing has make my life happier and better. I don't get in trouble like before and besides I am not ashamed because the FASD is not my fault."

— Bonnie

Diagnosis is important, because the earlier the intervention the more promising the outcome. It takes a toll out of the FASD individual and family if they must stumble through a very frustrating 5-10 years of searching before they receive the answer. With diagnosis we can respond differently, at least we have a map, given what we know in 2003 about FASD.

"It is important to get an accurate diagnosis as early as possible, an enriched family with lots of outside support and understanding."

— Louise

I would like to quote Bonnie Buxton, a Toronto journalist and advocate, co-founder of FAS World Canada, as she so gracefully sums up the situation. "We and our children need a great deal of help from the community, but most of the time our community fails us, and when our community fails us…it costs all of us dearly." (From her presentation "When did you Get the Tragedy of FASD," Bridging Communities Together)

In addition to an improved assessment tool, there needs to be increased awareness, communication and education about FASD

A Mother's Story: FAE Diagnosis is a Blessing

I have had my son Tim, since he was a baby. At that time I had already raised two of my own children, and had proved myself as a capable and loving parent. Equipped with my parenting knowledge and experience, I began my new journey with Tim, not expecting that it would differ drastically from raising my other children. By the time Tim was three, it grew clear to me that he was developing differently than his sister and brother.

Prior to the adoption I was informed of the possibility that Tim had been exposed to alcohol in uterine. I went through great frustration at the hands of professionals, teachers, doctors and social workers when I explained to them my concerns about Tim's bizarre behavior. They in turn assured me that I was overreacting and that nothing was wrong. Their reactions left me questioning my sanity. I kept bringing my FASD concerns into the conversation, but these concerns were promptly dismissed. I intuitively knew that the shallow answers I was given did not address the magnitude of the problem and their well-intended attempts to comfort me in turn made the situation worse, because it delayed our access to the services that could help Tim.

After 5 years of searching for answers, our frustration had reached a crest. Finally, a much-needed change came when Tim changed schools. He was about 8 at the time and entering grade three. Not long after Tim entered his new school, I received a phone call from his teacher. She expressed her concerns about how Tim was performing academically; apparently Tim was reading at below a grade one level. I was astounded by this news, as I had been assured by all of his previous teachers that he was doing very well in school, his reports cards were always good, no areas of weakness were listed. Finally we were able to address the issues that for so long had been dismissed. We began to meet individuals that would become a valuable support network for the next few years: an alert psychologist, an attentive principal and a doctor that specialized in addiction medicine. Each of these individuals contributed in shaping a plan for Tim's future. The psychologist offered aids to assist his learning as well as effective parenting techniques for me to employ. The need for structure, repetition and bundles of patience was the first parenting requirement. The medical doctor explained that it was as if certain areas of Tim's brain did not have the proper wiring, so certain areas lacked the ability to transmit information or store information. He explained the presence of something called "spotted memory syndrome," where the child will know information on a Monday and yet the following Thursday will remember absolutely nothing. Most importantly, the doctor stressed that Tim's misbehavior was not intentional, it was not a reflection of my failure nor was it a product of a flaw in his personality, rather it was caused by brain damage.

We were fortunate enough to have a school principal who was very knowledgeable about FASD and was both helpful and supportive of an individual plan for him within the regular class. The educational formula we used was for him to go to a special LA class consisting of only two students, four times a week, then also attend individual tutoring session for assistance with his reading skills. The teachers came on board and we organized regular meetings with my son, his teachers and principal, my husband and myself.

Finally we had received validation and an accurate diagnosis, with this our sanity returned. We finally knew what we were dealing with and how to cope with it. We were able to reframe Tim's secondary behaviors such as lying and stealing. We could see the picture with new vision, with a new understanding of his disabilities and were given new tools with which to deal with them. I had a renewed hope and a team of supporters to help the family. This team moved mountains. In grade three Tim could not read or write and had numerous behavioral barriers to becoming a successful graduate. I still remember with great pride how excited Tim was at the end of third grade when he received the most improved student award.

My son was diagnosed with FAE, which means he lacks the facial anomalies or any of the physical symptoms of the disease, but his brain and behavior are still affected.

John's Letter to the President of the United States

Dear Mr. and Mrs. Clinton,

My name is John Kellerman and I have Fetal Alcohol Syndrome. My mom is writing this for me, because I have a hard time writing letters. Even though my IQ is high enough to make me ineligible for state services (IQ 70 = one point too high to qualify), I can hardly sign my name, and I have been practicing for many years to do that. I also have a hard time with math and money, so I can't even go to the store. I am 21 years old and I cannot drive, because I could not pass the driver's test.

I just graduated from high school, and now I am starting my life in the adult world. But because of my disability, I cannot function as an adult. Even though I have the expressive language skills of an adult, and the body of an adult, I have the emotional development of a child, the conscience of a child, the social skills of a child. If you look at the research, you will realize this is all part of Fetal Alcohol Syndrome, and that I cannot progress in those areas in spite of my Mom and teachers working with me for many years.

Because I have Fetal Alcohol Syndrome, I need constant supervision. This is because the brain damage causes me to have trouble controling my impulses and inhibitions. I also have short memory problems. With lack of impulse control and poor judgment, I get into trouble easily and often, unless my Mom is nearby. This makes me frustrated and angry. I am afraid that I might get arrested some day, because of my poor impulse control. I'm afraid of what is going to happen to me when my Mom is not around to watch out for me.

Please help raise awareness about Fetal Alcohol Syndrome, so that we can prevent other kids from going through what I go through, and to get more services for people like me. Please proclaim September 9, 1999 as FAS AWARENESS DAY.

FAE, the Invisible Disability

Appropriately, FAE has been referred to as an "invisible disability." A study by Sampson, Streissguth, Bookstein and Barr addresses the categorization issue of FAS versus FAE or ARND. The data shows that patients diagnosed with FAS and others with FAE do not have meaningful behavioral differences, standardized scores of IQ, arithmetic and adaptive behaviors or secondary disabilities. In the case of FAE, a diagnosis is critical. As addressed by Anne Stressguith in her book, *Fetal Alcohol Syndrome: A Guide for Families and Communities*, individuals with FAE are more likely to be negatively impacted by secondary disabilities. Those who look completely normal but still have organic brain damage that affects their behavior are judged differently than those with visible symptoms of their disability. In the case of FAE, a child's misbehavior is often attributed to a flaw in their personality. If a child steals continuously, they are seen as bad individuals, their misbehavior is greeted with belligerence, anger and visible frustration by members of the community. When dealing with FAE, it can be even more critical that a diagnosis is in place, as with FAE the individual has no physical markers of the disorder and appears to be quite normal. The tragedy occurs when society's expectations of this FAE individual are normal, when it is impossible for the FAE individual to achieve this. Another example of the benefits of a label can be demonstrated when an FAE individual gets caught within the court system. He walks into a revolving door of re-offending due to the fact he looks "normal" and talks as if he is "normal," yet has no sense of consequence whatsoever.

One Family Shares their Story

Our tale begins 20 years ago. At that time we were operating an emergency medical receiving home for the foster care program. We took care of children who were considered difficult to place, many of which needed specialized medical care. One morning we got a call concerning a ten-week-old baby boy who had an emergency colostomy, and was to arrive directly from the hospital. He was a huge medical disaster, not only did he have a colostomy, but he had also developed severe allergies to all the colostomy medications as well as formula. At that time at only ten weeks, if you unsnapped his sleeper, he would go absolutely nuts because he knew that was a prelude to being hurt. Of course I did it to him all the time, because I needed to take care of him.

Time passed and he was developing into a gorgeous little baby. Then at 8 months he had to go to the hospital for another surgery to reconstruct the bowels, as they had prolapsed. So they took him back and closed up the colostomy and hooked him up the right way. They repaired him at eight months, put him back together and at that point he had an area worse than diaper rash, it was gruesome. At that time the judge decides that the birth family needed the opportunity to prove themselves. So he was removed from our home and placed with the family.

Eight months later I received a phone call that he was brought back into the hospital. He had bowel adhesions and he had been badly abused. I immediately went down to the hospital to see this little guy. When I arrived he was sitting in his high chair with his eyes squeezed shut. I leaned over and called his name. Upon hearing my voice he opened up his eyes, grabbed the tray on his high chair and ripped it right off. Then he leapt at me and clutched me as hard as he could. The nurses were shocked. According to the nurses, he had not moved since he arrived in the hospital. He never even budged. It was the most amazing experience. The little guy had new life in him. I then told the nurse to gather his clothes and belongings, I was taking him home. The nurse was baffled she did not know what to do with the situation. She told me that it was not possible without filling out the appropriate paper work. I replied, "if you do not want me to take that kid without permission, you better get on that phone." So she did. We were gone within an hour and now it is 17 years later. The sad thing is that he never lost any of that; all that abuse was still in him, it still affected him to this day.

It has been a long and hard journey. We were armed with a profound love for this child that we met 20 years ago, but there were many stuggles that tested the strength of our love. We knew from the beginning that our son had been exposed to alcohol in the womb and because of that he would be different than most children. We searched for answers and help in raising our child, but for the most part our questions went unanswered. So we learned through experience, through our calico past of failures and successes.

FAS Fallout

©2002 Teresa Kellerman

We know what the Primary Disabilities of FAS disorders are: small head and/or short stature, attention deficit disorder, physical anomalies like heart defects, reduced potential for intelligence, learning disabilities and behavior disorders. These are the physiological effects on the body and the brain caused directly by the exposure to alcohol during pregnancy. These are permanent, there is no cure.

The Secondary Conditions that are common among individuals with FAS disorders have been published by Ann Streissguth after years of studies. These occur as a result of the primary disabilities. They are often more serious in their effects on the individual, but they are totally preventable with early recognition and appropriate support services.

There is a third layer to the effects of prenatal exposure to alcohol. This is what I call FAS Fallout, the effects that are experienced by the families caring for the affected individuals, primarily the parents. The primary caretaker, usually the mother, is the one who is most seriously affected by FAS Fallout, but this can be experienced by the other spouse and by siblings and can have devastating results. The most common cause of FAS Fallout is lack of understanding by others about FAS disorders and lack of acceptance of the limitations imposed by the disorder and the restrictions needed to ensure safety and success for the child. There might also be alienation of siblings, friends, and extended family members. The divorce rate among these families is high.

Most often, the caregiver is an adoptive mother. In many cases, she adopted the child with the understanding that the child was healthy and normal. Sometimes the agency has withheld information about exposure prenatally to alcohol or other drugs for fear the child might not be accepted into the adoptive family. The result is a devastating grief over the loss of the dreams a parent has for a healthy, typical child.

When the caregiver is the birth mom, the primary pain is guilt. There is so much blame placed on the birth mother by society, that even when she did not intend to harm her child, even when she has won her struggle with addiction and is living a life clean and sober, she still fights off the combination of guilt, grief and fear.

Sometimes it is the birth father or a step mother who is raising the child. Sometimes the child is cared for by a foster family. There is often frustration, and unresolved anger toward the birth mother for exposing the child to alcohol before birth. The anger and the grief and the fear roll into a negative attitude that is hard to get past.

Something that is common for all the caregivers I have talked with is grief. There is a deep fear of the future. As the parent comes to realize the true nature of the FAS disorder (permanent brain damage rendering the child at high risk of never becoming totally independent), a shadow of fear overwhelms and sometimes consumes the parent. Outwardly, there is a great deal of anger, at the child, at the birth parent, at the system, at the alcohol, at the alcohol industry, at the world that does not understand or accept their child. The grief is universal. If the fear and anger are not allowed to surface, there may be great sadness and depression. Most parents cycle through all of these feelings, over and over. And for parents of children with FAS disorders, the grief is heavier than for most parents of children with other disorders. The stress is beyond what a normal person is expected to cope with.

The results of FAS Fallout for the family include: chronic depression that needs to be treated with anti-depressants and therapy; social isolation, temptation to self medicate with alcohol; chronic fatigue and burnout. What can extended family and community members and helping professionals do to minimize FAS Fallout for the primary caregiver? What are the intervention strategies that can be offered to help ensure success for the family? Let's fight Fallout with Fallout!

Friendship, or at least feelings of empathy

Acceptance of the reality of FAS

Listen to the ones who really understand

Learn about FAS disorders

Organize to take action

Understand the nature of FAS behaviors

Talk to everyone to raise awareness

Friendship in dark times and in crisis, as well as when things are going well. Call or visit, and offer help, even if it is just a shoulder to cry on or an ear to listen to the latest crisis, even if it's the same crisis over and over. Bring laughter and love and maybe some affection. A hug from someone who really cares is priceless.

Acceptance of the reality of FAS. The child has gifts and talents, recognize them. The child has limitations imposed by the FAS disorders. You can help by not dismissing the disorder by referring to it as a stage they will grow out of, or saying things like "All kids are like that." Not all kids have inconsistent ability to control their impulses, poor judgment, and emotional development of a child half their chronological age.

Listen to the parents. They are the ones who know FAS best. They understand the child and know best what their child needs to succeed.

Learn about FAS disorders. Read the materials the parents give you. Attend a class or conference on FAS. Ask questions. Learn to think differently, with an open mind.

Organize and take action. Offer to help form a non-profit community group. The emotional organization they need is a support group. If there is not a local group to attend, help to form one. There are many Internet groups that offer daily support, understanding and solutions to common problems. Parents also need freedom from the chaos in their lives and homes. The physical chaos of homes of these families seems to be a common occurrence. The answer to this can be found on the Internet as well, at www.FlyLady.Net. This is a good place for moms to start to put their lives back together. If the family does not have a computer and/or Internet access, this would be the ideal first step to providing some real help to the family. First stop: www.fasstar.com.

Understand the true nature of FAS disorders. The behavior problems are due primarily to brain damage from alcohol, not necessarily poor parenting. Most parents have been suspected or accused of sexual abuse or human rights violations. All children with FAS disorders exhibit inappropriate sexual behaviors. All children with FAS disorders need restrictions that would be considered unfair or unethical if imposed on typical children. Refrain from judgment until you get to know the family well and learn all the details behind the issues.

Talk to everyone you know about FAS disorders. Tell them everything you are learning. Tell them about the family's experiences (maintaining confidentiality, of course). Talk to your legislators and policymakers, and let them know what the families need and what the community needs as well (funding for services, public education, teacher training, etc.). Raising awareness in the world begins with one person – you, right there in your own family and your own neighborhood. Talk about alcohol and addiction. Give a talk about FAS to a local civic group, or at a health class at a local school. Talk to your hairdresser, your delivery person, your spouse, your third cousin twice removed. The greater the awareness, the better the chance to begin finding solutions. Take part in the next FAS Awareness

Day event. If one is not already planned, then plan one. Get ideas at www.fasworld.com. This is the kind of thing that the parents are doing all on their own, that they would really appreciate some help with.

If for each stressed out parent there was just one dedicated friend who would be willing to carry out these intervention strategies, then FAS Fallout would slowly disappear, and in its place we would see Fun and Freedom instead.

References

Abel, Ernest L. (1995). "An Update on Incidence of FAS: FAS is not an Equal Opportunity Birth Defect." *Neurotoxicology and Teratology*: 437-43.

Abel, Ernest. (1988). "Fetal Alcohol in Families." *Neurotoxicology and Teratology*. 10:1-2.

Abkarian, G.G. (1992). "Communication Effects of Prenatal Alcohol Exposure." *Journal of Communication Disorders*. 25: 221-240.

Barr, H.M., Streissguth, A.P., Darby, B.L., Sampson, P.D. (1990). "Prenatal exposure to alcohol, caffeine, tobacco and aspirin: Effects on fine and gross motor performance in four year old children." *Development Psychology*. 26: 339-348.

Becker, Howard C. et al. (1994). "Animal Research: Charting the Course for FAS." *Alcohol Health and Research World*. 18.1:10-16.

Browne, Annette, et al. (1998). *Women and Alcohol: Assessment, Women-Centered Perspectives and Treatment*. Prince George: University of Northern British Columbia.

Burd, Larry, et al. (1999). "The FAS Screen: A Rapid Screening Tool for Fetal Alcohol Syndrome." *Addiction Biology*. 4: 329-336.

Burd, Larry, et al. (2000). "Screening for Fetal Alcohl Syndrome: Is it Feasible and Necessary?" *Addiction Biology*. 5: 127-139.

Burgess, D. & Streissguth, A. (1992). "Fetal Alcohol Syndrome and Fetal Alcohol Effect: Principles for Educators." *Phi Delta Kappan*. 74; 24-30.

Buxton, Bonnie. (2003, 28 May). *When Did You "Get" the Tragedy of FASD?* FASSTAR. http://www.come-over.to/FAS/getfasd.htm.

Conry, Julianne & Fast, Diane. (2000). *FAS and the Criminal Justice System*. Vancouver: British Columbia Fetal Alcohol Syndrome Resource Society.

Conry, Julianne, Fast, Diane and Loocke, C. (1999). "Identifying FAS Among Youth in the Criminal Justice System." *Juvenile Developmental Behavioural Pediatirics*. 20: 370-372.

Chernoff, G.F. (1977). "The Fetal Alcohol Syndrome in Mice: An Animal Model." *Teratology*. 15(3): 223-229.

Donovan, C.P. (1991). "Factors Predisposing, Enabling and Reinforcing Routine Screening Patients for Preventing Fetal Alcohol Syndrome: A Survey of New Jersey Physicians." *Journal of Drug Education*. 21(1): 35-42.

Fleming, Michael. (1999). *Identification and Care of Fetal Alcohol-Exposed Children: A Guide for Primary-Care Providers*. Rockville: NIAAA Publication.

Golden, Janet. (2000). "A Tempest in a Cocktail Glass: Mothers, Alcohol and Television, 1977-1996." *Journal of Health, Politics and Law*. 25, 3:473-498.

Graefe, Sara. (1999). *Parenting Children Affected by Fetal Alcohol Syndrome: A Guide for Daily Living*. Vancouver: Society of Special Needs Adoptive Parents.

Huebert, Kathy, and Cindy Raftis. (1996). *Fetal alcohol Syndrome and other Alcohol Related Birth Defects*. Edmonton: AADAC Resource Development and Marketing.

Jones, K.L. & Smith, D.W. (1973). "Recognition of the Fetal Alcohol Syndrome in early infancy." *Lancet*. 2: 999-1001.

Jones, K.L. & Smith, D.W. (1975). "The Fetal Alcohol Syndrome." *Teratology*. 12: 1-10.

Kapp, Frances & O' Malley, Kieran. (2001). *Watch for the Rainbows: True Stories for Educators and other Caregivers of Children with FASD*. Calgary: Francis Kapp Education.

Kaskutas, Lee Ann & Graves, Karen. (2001). "Pre-pregnancy Drinking: How Drink Size Affects Risk Assessment." *Addiction*. 96: 1199-1209.

Kent, Heather. (2000). "MD Helped Bring Fetal Alcohol Syndrome Out of the Closet in BC." *Canadian Medical Association Journal*. 162, 9: 1388-89.

Kleinfled, Judith & Siobhan Westcott, eds. (1993). *Fantastic Antone Succeeds: Adolescents and Adults with FAS*. Fairbanks: University of Alaska Press.

Lancaster, F.E. (1994). "Alcohol and White Matter Development A Review." *Alcoholism: Clinical and Experimental Research*. 18: 644-647.

Legge, Carole, Roberts, Gary & Butler, Mollie. (2001). *Situational Analysis: Fetal Alcohol Syndrome/Fetal Alcohol Effects and the Effects of Other Substance Use During Pregnancy*. Ottawa: Health Canada.

Lemoine, P.H., Harousseau, J., Borteyru, J.P. and Mennet, J.C. (1968). "Children of Alcoholic Parents: Abnormalities Observed in 127 Cases." *Quest Medical*. 21: 476-492.

McLean, Candis. (2000). "The Fetal Alcohol Crisis." *Alberta Report*. 27, 10: 32-36.

Macionis, John. (2002). *Sociology*. Toronto: Pearson Education Canada Inc.

Malbin, Diane. (1993). *Fetal Alcohol Syndrome/ Fetal Alcohol Effects: Strategies for Professionals*. Center City: Hazelden.

Mayer, Lorna, ed. (1999). *Living and Working with Fetal Alcohol Syndrome/Effects*. Winnipeg: Interagency FAS/E Program.

McCreight, Brenda. (1997). *Recognizing and Managing Children with Fetal Alcohol Syndrome/Fetal Alcohol Effect: A Guidebook*. Washington, DC: CWLA Press.

Raftis, Sara & Reynolds, Wendy. (1996). *Give and Take: A Booklet for Pregnant Women about Alcohol and other drugs*. Kingston: AWARE Press.

Ratcliff, Kathryn. (2002). *Women and Health: Power, Technology, Inequality, and Conflict in a Gendered World*. Boston: Allyn & Bacon.

Roberts, Gary & Nanson, Jo. (2001). *Best Practices: Fetal Alcohol Syndrome, Fetal Alcohol Effect and the Effects of Other substance Use During Pregnancy*. Ottawa, Health Canada.

Roth, Paula, ed. (1991). *Alcohol and Drugs are Women's Issues*. London: The

Scarecrow Press.

Sandmaier, Marian. (1992). *The Invisible Alcoholic: Women and Alcohol.* Bradenton: TAB Books.

Schmidt, G. & Turpin, J. (1999). *Fetal Alcohol Syndrome: Effect and Developing a Community Response.* Halifax, NS: Fernwood Press.

Smitherman, C. (1994). "The Lasting impact of Fetal Alcohol Syndrome and Fetal Alcohol Effect on Children and Adolescents." *Journal of Pediatric Health Care.* 8 (1): 121-126.

Stratton, K., Howe, C. and Battagliaf, F.C. (1996). *Fetal Alcohol Syndrome: Diagnosis, Epidemiology, Prevention and Treatment.* Washington National Academy Press.

Streissguth, A. (1996). *Understanding the Occurrence of Secondary Disabilities in Clients with FAS/FAE.* Final Report Available from the Fetal Alcohol and Drug Unit Seattle Washington.

Streissguth, A.P. (1997). *Fetal Alcohol Syndrome: A Guide for Families and Communities.* Baltimore, Maryland: Paul H. Brookes Publishing Company.

Streissguth, A.P., Aase, J.M., Clarren, S.K., Randalls, S.P., LaDue, R.A., Smith, D.A. (1991). "Fetal Alcohol Syndrome in Adolescents and Adults." *Journal of American Medical Association.* 265(15): 1961-1967.

Streissguth, A.P., Barr, H.M., Press, S. (1996). "A Fetal Alcohol Behavioral Scale for Describing Children and Adults Effected by Prenatal Exposure." *Alcoholism: Clinical and Experimental Research.* 20(2): 73a.

Streissguth, A.P. (1999). *The Challenge of Fetal Alcohol Syndrome: Overcoming Secondary Disabilities.* University of Washington Press.

Warren, Kenneth, and Laurie Foudin. (2001). "Alcohol-Related Birth Defects – Past, Present and Future." *Alcohol Research and Health.* 25, 3:153-158.

Waterson, Jan. (2000). *Women and Alcohol in Social Context: Mother's Ruin Revisited.* New York: Palgrave.

Internet References

Alcohol Alert
  http://www.drugs.indiana.edu/publications/ncadi/alerts/html

Justice and Sentencing 1994
  http://www.ombud.gov.bcca/publications/reports/html

Yukon Physicians now required to report FAS
  http://www.gov.uk.ca/news/2000/octoberoo/oo/90.pdf

Fetal Alcohol Syndrome: Implications for Corrections Services
  http://www.csc.scc.qc.ca/text/rsrch/reports/r71/r71e.html

National Crime Prevention

http://www.web.apc.org/npc

FAS and Prisons
http://www.arbi.org/courthos/html

This is the home page of Alcohol-related Birth Injury (FASD) Resource Site and offers information about FAS and ARBIs as well as links for many related sites.
http://www.arbi.org

This is the homepage of Canadian Center on Substance Abuse (CCSA) for information regarding alcohol and drug abuse.
http://www.ccsa.ca
The FAS/FAE Information Service at www.ccsa.ca/fasgen.htm provides a directory of FAS/FAE Information and Support Services in Canada.

http://www.come-over.to/FAS

http://www.come-over.to/FASCRC

http://www.fasbookshelf.com

An organization and information on FAS in french (Quebec)
http://www.safera.qc.ca

FAS/E support network of BC
http://www.fetalalcohol.com

FAS Link
http://www.acbr.com/fas

Your source for evidence-based information about the safety or risk of drugs, chemicals and disease during pregnancy and lactation.
http://www.motherisk.org

This is the website of Alberta Family & Social Services where additional information on services provided by this department may be found. The AF&SS website provides updated information on government services as well as information links to resources on FASD and the interprovincial FASD partnership with Saskatchewan and Manitoba.
http://www.gov.ab.ca and http://www.child.gov.ab.ca
Look under Programs and Services for a complete description of the provincial FASD initiative or go to the website at:
http://www.acs.gov.ab.ca/fas/index.html

Community Directory

Toll Free Information Services

FAS/FAE Information Service:

Call toll-free: 1-800-559-4514 for bilingual information on fetal alcohol spectrum disorder. This service is provided by the Canadian Center of Substance Abuse (CCSA), through its National Clearinghouse on Substance Abuse, with additional funding from Health Canada and the Brewers' Association of Canada.

Alcohol and Substance Abuse Helpline:

Call toll-free: 1-877-327-4636 for answers to questions on the use of alcohol and other substances during pregnancy and breast-feeding. Provided by the Motherisk program of The Hospital for Sick Children, Toronto, the helpline is designed for women in regions where convenient access to medical care is difficult. Where possible, callers will be referred to additional resources and support programs in the caller's area. The service is bilingual and confidential, as well as Canada-wide and toll-free. 9-5 in every time zone.

National Organizations

FAS/FAE Information Service
Canadian Centre on Substance Abuse (CCSA)

300 - 75 Albert Street
Ottawa, ON K1P 5E7
Tel: 1-800-559-4514 (toll free in Canada) (613) 235-4048, ext. 223
Fax: (613) 235-8101
Email: fas@ccsa.ca URL: www.ccsa.ca/fasgen.htm

Services: Through its National Clearinghouse on Substance Abuse, information resources are provided in answer to individual requests through the 1-800 number, fax, email and written request.

FASworld Canada

Ms. Bonnie Buxton/Brian Philcox, Founders
1509 Danforth Avenue
Toronto, ON M4J 5C3
Tel: (416) 465-7766 Fax: (416) 465-8890
Email: fasworldcanada@rogers.com
URL: www.fasworld.com

Services: FASworld Canada is a pro-active, non-profit organization which strives to dramatically reduce the incidence of fetal alcohol disorders, reduce the incidence of secondary disabilities among individuals living with mental or physical damage caused by maternal drinking in pregnancy and to assist families and caregivers of people with fetal alcohol spectrum disorder (FASD). FASworld Canada works with health units, family support groups and other interested organizations who form the chapter network in communities across the country. Individuals and groups are invited to apply for membership or chapter status.

Health Canada, FAS/FAE Team

Ms. Mary Johnston, Manager
Division of Childhood and Adolescence
Room C967, Jeanne Mance Building
Tunney's Pasture, Postal Locator: 1909C2
Ottawa, ON K1A 1B4
Tel: (613) 946-1779 Fax: (613) 946-2324
Email: mary_johnston@hc-sc.gc.ca
URL: www.healthcanada.ca/fas

Services: In 1999, funding of $11 million over three years was allocated to enhance activities related to: Public Awareness and Education, FAS/FAE Training and Capacity Development, Early Identification and Diagnosis, Coordination, Integration of Services, Surveillance, and a Strategic Project Fund. Health Canada's Division of Childhood and Adolescence role is to implement activities outlined in the initiative.

Alberta Partnership on Fetal Alcohol Syndrome

Alberta Family & Social Services co-chairs the Alberta Partnership on FAS with the Alberta Alcohol and Drug Abuse Commission. The purpose of this alliance of partners is to develop, promote and coordinate a provincial plan for the prevention/intervention, care and support of FAS/ARBD-affected individuals.

Contact Darren Joslin at (780) 415-0523

For more information, see http://www.acs.gov.ab.ca/fas/index.html

Well Community-Well Families Finding Solutions to Fetal Alcohol Syndrome

Collaborative Community Project of Health For 2, Bissell Center and Success by 6
10527-96 Street
Edmonton, AB
T5H 2H6
Contact: The Bissell Center
(780) 423-2285 Fax (780) 429-7908

Well Community-Well Families is a multi-level community development program aimed at building the capacity of Central Edmonton communities to support healthy pregnancies and families.

Goals are:

To increase awareness of FASD in Central Edmonton among community residents, agencies and organizations.

To empower women who are at high risk of having a child with FASD.

To strengthen the capacity of informal and formal community resources to address and prevent FASD.

To empower adults with FASD to make and maintain positive changes.

First Steps- Prevention Program for FASD

A program of Catholic Social Services
#223 Abbottsfield Mall
Edmonton, AB
Program Manager: Mary Berube
(780) 477-1999 Fax (780) 477-2499

First Steps is a program of Catholic Social Services. The First Steps program was initiated to help women who are at risk of giving birth to a child with FASD.

Goals are:

To reduce future births of children with FASD.

To ensure children are in safe and stable environments

To support parents to build and maintain healthy, independent families.

Coaching Families FASD Family Intervention Program

A program of Catholic Social Services
#223 Abbottsfield Mall
Edmonton, AB
Program Manager: Mary Berube
(780) 477-1999 Fax (780) 477-2499

Coaching Families is a pilot project to help families who have children with FASD. The program provides intensive support for 3-6 months to help access services for diagnosis where appropriate, provide tools and strategies for adjustment in living with children with FASD, and make referrals to counseling services and parenting supports.

Step by Step

A program of Catholic Social Services
#223 Abbottsfield Mall
Edmonton, AB
Program Manager: Mary Berube
(780) 477-1999 Fax (780) 477-2499

Mentor program for mothers who have FASD and who are parenting children. We provide support, home visiting and advocacy by offering/helping the client:

- Access and integrate parenting information
- Stabilize financial matters
- Access health care and immunizations
- Access counseling services, as required
- Improve relationships with schools, etc.
- Connect with other community resources

Mentoring Case Management Pilot Project

Serving individuals affected by FASD from the ages of 16-24. There are two case managers, one in the Spruce Grove, Stony Plain, Evansburg area and the other in the Jasper, Hinton, Edson area.

Contact:
Region 8 East Case Manager
Rebecca Wiens
Spruce Grove Child and Family Services Center
#200, 131 - Avenue
Spruce Grove, AB
T7X 2Z8
Rebecca.Wiens@gov.ab.ca

Elves Child Development Center

Elves Early Education Program provides intensive early intervention for children with FASD from a transdisciplinary approach. Within our format, complex tasks are broken down into small steps and repeatedly presented to the child with positive consequences for appropriate behaviors. These procedures are applied and embedded within a developmental play-based curriculum. Admission criteria and program information can be obtained by contacting the social worker at (780) 454-5310.

10421-159 Street
Edmonton, AB
T5P 3AG

Alberta Aboriginal Committee on FAS/FAE

Ms. Ruth Morin - Chief Executive Officer
Nechi Training Research and Health Promotions Institute
Box 34007, Kingsway Mall P.O.
Edmonton, AB T5G 3G4
Tel: (780) 459-1884; 1-800-459-1884 (toll free in Alberta)
Fax: (780) 458-1883
Email: ruth-morin@nechi.com

Services: This Committee was struck to ensure the Aboriginal perspective receives consideration, recognition and respect in all matters related to FAS/FAE. Its purposes are to focus on primary prevention, intervention, care and support in a culturally appropriate manner, working in concert with provincial and national stakeholders to harmonize traditional Aboriginal principles and conventional (mainstream) principles to educate and heal.

Alberta Ministry of Children's Services

Ms. Cynthia Farmer - Co-chair
Alberta Partnership on Fetal Alcohol Syndrome
5th Floor, Sterling Place
9940 - 106 Street
Edmonton, AB T5K 2N2
Tel: (780) 422-5680 Fax: (780) 422-5415
Email: cynthia.farmer@gov.ab.ca

Services: Also co-chaired by Alberta Alcohol and Drug Abuse Commission, the mandate of the Alberta Partnership on FAS, is to develop, promote and coordinate a comprehensive, culturally sensitive, provincial plan for the prevention, intervention, and care and support of individuals with fetal alcohol syndrome or alcohol related birth defects.

Alberta Partnership on Fetal Alcohol Syndrome

Ms. Diane Lamb - Project Manager
AADAC Enhanced Services for Women
210 - 10909 Jasper Avenue
Edmonton, AB T5J 3M9
Tel: (780) 422-3055 Fax: (780) 422-5237
Email: diane.lamb@aadac.gov.ab.ca

Services: Also co-chaired by Alberta Ministry of Children's Services, the mandate of the Alberta Partnership, through the FAS Committee, is to develop, promote and coordinate a comprehensive, culturally sensitive, provincial plan for the prevention, intervention, and care and support of individuals with FAS or alcohol-related birth defects.

Children's Services

Ms. Donna Debolt
124 Coachwood Point
Lethbridge, AB T1K 6A8
Tel: (403) 381-5673 Fax: (403) 381-2005
Email: donna.debolt@gov.ab.ca

Services: Donna is working with the Alberta Partnership on Fetal Alcohol Syndrome in building a comprehensive provincial plan for the prevention, intervention, care and support of FAS/ARND-affected individuals. As an FAS/E Specialist, she is assisting with the development of a provincial strategic plan, assisting communities with building community capacity and has an ongoing role in advocacy and case management support.

FAS/ARND Employability Specialist

Mr. Brian Mader
Canada/Alberta Service Centre West
#120 - 15710 87 Avenue
Edmonton, AB T5R 5W9
Tel: (780) 422-2603 Fax: (780) 422-0745
Email: brian.mader@gov.ab.ca

Services: The Centre provides training and employment options as well as case management services for youth and adults. Occasionally the Centre refers clients for psychological assessment and diagnostic testing.

FAS Association

Ms. Florence McIntyre Palmer - Coordinator
603 Mariposa Place NE
Calgary, AB T2E 5V9
Tel: (403) 276-1577

Services: This is an FAS support group, for parents and professionals, providing information on a wide range of concerns and questions on FAS/FAE. The Association has produced a book entitled *Two Sides of the Coin.*

FAS Consultant

Ms. Marilyn Frye - Parent/Mentor
Box 3533
Wainwright, AB T9W 1T5
Tel: (780) 842-2802; 1-866-842-5585 (toll-free in Alberta only)
Fax: (780) 842-5987
Email: mfrye@telusplanet.net

Services: To consult with communities and families and to promote awareness by workshops and discuss solutions in response to Fetal Alcohol Syndrome Disorder. To support and create parent support groups to build a network for families to access is another service.

Marilyn has presented at many conferences and workshops across the country.

FAS Coordinating Committee, Region 1

Ms. Hazel Mitchell - Program Administrator
Lethbridge Community College
3000 College Drive South
Lethbridge, AB T1K 1L6
Tel: (403) 329-7200 Fax: (403) 317-3542
Email: hazel.mitchell@lethbridgecollege.ab.ca

Services: The Committee was established in the city of Lethbridge in 1991. It identifies community needs and assists with coordination of FAS efforts in the areas of prevention, resource development, support to FAS/FAE individuals and their caregivers, and public and professional education and undertakes activities within the community to support the provincial plan for the prevention, intervention and care of individuals and families affected by FAS or alcohol-related birth defects.

FAS Coordinating Committee, Region 2

Ms. Linda Langevin
Palliser Health Authority
666 - 5th Street SW
Medicine Hat, AB T1A 4H6
Tel: (403) 528-8146
Email: llangevin@pha.ab.ca

Services: The regional FAS Committee coordinates and undertakes activities within the community to support the provincial plan for the prevention, intervention and care of individuals and families affected by FAS or alcohol related birth defects.

FAS Coordinating Committee, Region 5

Ms. Trina Butchart
c/o Big Country Outreach Program
P.O. Box 2547
Drumheller, AB T0J 0Y0
Tel: (403) 823-0442 Fax: (403) 823-2446
Email: tbutchart@hotmail.com

Services: The regional FAS Committee coordinates and undertakes activities within the community to support the provincial plan for the prevention, intervention and care of individuals and families affected by FAS or alcohol-related birth defects.

FAS Coordinating Committee, Region 8

Ms. Sheona Ayles - Early Intervention Coordinator
Hinton Health Unit - Westview Regional Health Authority
1280A Switzer Drive
Hinton, AB T7V 1T5
Tel: (780) 865-2277; (780) 865-6249 (cell) Fax: (780) 865-3727
Email: sheona.ayles@westviewrha.ab.ca

Services: The regional FAS Committee coordinates and undertakes activities within the community to support the provincial plan for the prevention, intervention and care of individuals and families affected by FAS or alcohol related birth defects.

FAS Coordinating Committee, Region 9

Mr. Kyle Archer
Community Services Unit
County of Wetaskiwin Building
Wetaskiwin, AB T9A 2G1
Tel: (780) 361-1388 Fax: (780) 361-1361
Email: kyle.archer@gov.ab.ca

Services: The regional FAS Committee coordinates and undertakes activities within the community to support the provincial plan for the prevention, intervention and care of individuals and families affected by FAS or alcohol related birth defects.

FAS Coordinating Committee, Region 16

Ms. Valerie Crowe
Fort McMurray Association for Community Living
9915 Franklin Avenue
Fort McMurray, AB T9H 2K4
Tel: (780) 791-3009 Fax: (780) 791-7506
Email: valcrowe@shawlink.ca

Services: The regional FAS Committee coordinates and undertakes activities within the community to support the provincial plan for the prevention, intervention and care of individuals and families affected by FAS or alcohol related birth defects.

FAS Coordinating Committee, Region 17

Mr. Gerry Cyr
Alberta Alcohol and Drug Abuse Commission
P.O. Box 632
9813 - 102nd Street
High Level, AB T0H 1Z0
Tel: (780) 926-2265
Email: gerry.cyr@aadac.gov.ab.ca

Services: The regional FAS Committee coordinates and undertakes activities within the community to support the provincial plan for the prevention, intervention and care of individuals and families affected by FAS or alcohol related birth defects.

FASD Support Program, Region 9

Ms. Winnie Wong - Program Manager
Catholic Social Services
4715 - 50 Avenue
Wetaskiwin, AB T9A 0R9
Tel: (780) 352-5535 Fax: (780) 352-3190
Email: winnie.wong@catholicsocialservices.ab.ca
URL: www.catholicsocialservices.ab.ca

Services: Transition Support Workers provide support and intervention to affected clients and families in the form of referral to community resources, education, behavioral strategies, and intervention at school and work.

FAS/FAE and Related Birth Disorders Support Group

Lethbridge, AB
Tel: Shirley: (403) 320-1490; Pat: (403) 327-1147; Mary: (403) 381-4640; Jackie: (403) 327-7429

Services: This group was established to provide support, understanding and education for families with children affected by prenatal exposure to drugs or alcohol through referrals, education to individuals or groups, residential placement, housing and vocational employment information, parental support teams, and training to educators.

FAS/FAE Support Group

Ms. Alice McNeil
c/o Adoption 2000 Consulting
Regional Resource Centre
631 Prospect Drive SW
Medicine Hat, AB T1A 4C2
Tel: (403) 529-8079 Fax: (403) 528-8147
Email: adopfost@telusplanet.net

Services: A support group for parents and caregivers is held on the second Tuesday of the month throughout the year. Other services provided to families and children include family mediation, counselling and behavior management.

FAS Steering Committee, Region 4

Mr. Russell Moore - Addiction Counsellor
AADAC Adult Counselling and Prevention Services
Stevenson Building, 2nd floor
1177 - 11th Avenue South West
Calgary, AB T2R 0G5
Tel: (403) 297-3075 Fax: (403) 297-3036
Email: Russ.Moore@aadac.gov.ab.ca

Services: The regional FAS Committee coordinates and undertakes activities within the community to support the provincial plan for the prevention, intervention and care of individuals and families affected by FAS or alcohol related birth defects.

FASD Family Advocacy and Parent Mentorship Projects

Ms. Diane Wrubleski
#208, 223 12 Avenue SW
Calgary, AB T2R 0G9
Tel: (403) 263-3447 Fax: (403) 202-7254
Email: jffas@telusplanet.net

Services: Both projects are for families or individuals aged 0-30 years. No referrals necessary. The FASD Family Advocacy Project provides professionals trained in areas of human services who work with the family and in each family's community to help consolidate community professionals connected with the family into an FASD-informed team. The FASD Parent Mentorship Project offers in-home parent-to-parent support to families affected by FASD. Parent Mentors who are parents or long-time caregivers of children affected by FASD work with the parents to provide emotional support, validation and encouragement in parenting a child with FASD.

FASS - Fetal Alcohol Support Society

Thelma Vincent
Grande Prairie, AB
Tel: (780) 814-7624
Email: thelmant@telusplanet.net

Services: The objectives of FASS are to promote and facilitate education, prevention, intervention, diagnosis and/or assessment, care and supports from birth to death of persons affected by Fetal Alcohol; to promote and facilitate support groups for caregivers and those persons who may be affected by Fetal Alcohol; and to provide necessary equipment materials, space, furniture and personnel to carry out the objectives of the Society. Support meetings are held the 2nd and 4th Thursday of each month, at 7:30 p.m. at the Schubert Building (ILS boardroom) in Grande Prairie. For support, you may also contact Lorraine: 532-3726 or John & Sharon: 539-5651.

First Steps Program and Coaching Families, FASD Interventionists

Ms. Mary (Vandenbrink) Berube - Program Manager/FASD Specialist
Catholic Social Services/Ministry of Childrens Services
223 Abbotsford Mall
3210 - 118 Avenue
Edmonton, AB T5W 4W1
Tel: (780) 477-1999 ext. 231
Email: mary.berube@catholicsocialservices.ab.ca

Services: Mary Berube (formerly Vandenbrink), BSW, RSW, is an FASD Specialist for Children's Services who also works as Program Manager of First Steps, Birth to Three and Coaching Families, FASD Interventionists with Catholic Social Services. First Steps is a program for birth mothers at high risk for combining pregnancy with drug and alcohol use. Coaching Families is a program that places mentors/coaches within families to support them as they live with a family member that has FASD.

Joining Forces - Fetal Alcohol Society

#208, 223 - 12 Avenue SW
Calgary, AB T2R 0G9
Tel: (403) 202-7233 Fax: (403) 202-7254
Email: jffas@telusplanet.net

Services: This is a non-profit society formed to enhance the well-being of individuals and families affected by fetal alcohol. Caregiver support meetings are held every second and fourth Thursday of the month from 7:00 to 9:00 p.m. There are two programs available for families or individuals aged 0-30: the FASD Family Advocacy Project provides professionals trained in areas of human services who work with the family and the community to help consolidate community professionals involved with the family into an FASD-informed team; the FASD Parent Mentorship Project offers in-home parent-to-parent support to families. Mentors work with the parents to provide emotional support, validation and encouragement in parenting a child with FASD. Referrals are not necessary.

Lakeland FAS Committee (Region 12 Health Authority)

Ms. Sue Lysachok - Chair
Audrey McFarlane, Program Coordinator
c/o Lakeland Centre for FAS
Box 479
Cold Lake, AB T9M 1P1
Tel: (780) 594-9905 Fax: (780) 594-9907
Email: sue.lysachok@aadac.gov.ab.ca

Services: The Regional Committee coordinates and undertakes activities to increase awareness of and prevent FAS. Two multi-disciplinary, mobile, diagnostic teams provide diagnosis for children and adults throughout the region. A team of staff provide follow-up support to individuals and families affected as well as training about FAS and best-practices, to professionals and paraprofessionals. A staff member provides intensive mentoring and support to high-risk pregnant women, assisting them to achieve and maintain sobriety in order to prevent an FAS birth.

Lethbridge Family Services, DaCapo

Ms. Brenda Cannady
1107 - 2nd Avenue A North
Lethbridge, AB T1H 0E6

Tel: (403) 320-9119 Fax: (403) 329-4924
Email: bcannady@lethbridge-family-services.com URL: www.lethbridge-family-services.com

Services: The agency provides residential, day program and/or vocational services for FAS/FAE individuals which focus on stability, structure, routine and long-term placements. Telephone support is available to individuals requiring information about FAS/FAE.

Peace Region FAS Committee

Ms. Wendy Ayele - Committee Chair
Peace Health Region
Bag 400
Peace River, AB T8S 1T6
Tel: (780) 624-7253 Fax: (780) 624-7255
Email: erin.harris@gov.ab.ca

Services: The regional FAS Committee coordinates and undertakes activities within the community to support the provincial plan for the prevention, intervention and care of individuals and families affected by FAS or alcohol related birth defects.

Physician/Psychiatrist Dr. Kieran D. O'Malley

#200 - 2003 14th Street NW
Calgary, AB T2M 3N4
Tel: (403) 289-0388 Fax: (403) 255-4406
Email: kieranom@shaw.ca; kieranom@u.washington.edu

Services: Dr. O'Malley has a special interest in FASD (fetal alcohol spectrum disorders) and psychiatric disorders of children and adolescents. He is involved with the Fetal Alcohol and Drug Unit in Seattle and the FASD community. He is teaching and doing research on FASD with the University of Washington Department of Psychiatry and Behavioral Sciences, offers psychiatric consultation to patients previously diagnosed with FASD and has a community psychiatry consultation practice in Calgary dealing with Fetal Alcohol Spectrum Disorder and Austistic Spectrum Disorder patients (children, adolescents and young adults).

Region 6 Fetal Alcohol Syndrome Committee

Ms. Shirley Gibson - Chairperson
Alberta Alcohol and Drug Abuse Commission

Main Floor, Provincial Building
4920 - 52nd Street
Red Deer, AB T4N 6K8
Tel: (403) 340-7030 Fax: (403) 340-4804
Email: shirley.gibson@aadac.gov.ab.ca

Services: The regional FAS Committee coordinates and undertakes activities within the community to support the provincial plan for the prevention, intervention and care of individuals and families affected by FAS or alcohol-related birth defects.

Region 10 FASD Steering Committee

Ms. Mary Ellen Jackson-Herman
AADAC Adult Services
10010 - 102 A Avenue
Edmonton, AB T5J 3G2
Tel: (780) 415-0036 Fax: (780) 427-4180
Email: maryellen.j-herman@aadac.gov.ab.ca

Services: The Regional FASD Committee coordinates and plans activities within the community to support the provincial plan for the prevention, intervention and care of individuals and families affected by FASD.

WJS Alberta

Mr. Peter Farnden - Regional Director
#218 - 10509 81 Avenue
Edmonton, AB T6E 1X7
Tel: (780) 439-5087 Fax: (780) 431-2196
Email: pfarnden@wjsgroup.com

Services: WJS Alberta provides specific service to individuals with FAS including residential, outreach, behavioral assessment and program design. Services are located throughout Northern Alberta from Edmonton north. You may also contact Heather Dowhaluk, Tel: (780) 657-3307; Fax: (780) 657-3309; Email: hfraessdowhaluk@wjs-group.com OR Barb Chaffee, Tel: (780) 674-3664; Fax: (780) 674-3806; Email: bchaffee@wjsgroup.com.

Working Together for FAS/E, Region 11

Mr. Garry Sebulsky
2nd Floor, Pembina Professional Centre

#210 - 1004 107th Street
Westlock, AB T7P 2K0
Tel: (780) 349-5478 Fax: (780) 349-5603
Email: children.services11@gov.ab.ca; garry.sebulsky@gov.ab.ca

Services: The regional FAS Committee coordinates and undertakes activities within the community to support the provincial plan for the prevention, intervention and care of individuals and families affected by FAS or alcohol-related birth defects.

British Columbia

The Asante Centre for Fetal Alcohol Syndrome

Ms. Audrey Salahub - Coordinator
22326 (A) McIntosh Avenue
Maple Ridge, BC V2X 3C1
Tel: (604) 467-7101; 1-866-327-7101 (toll free in Canada) Fax: (604) 467-7102
Email: info@asantecentre.org URL: www.asantecentre.org

Services: This is a diagnostic, assessment and family support centre for individuals of all ages affected by fetal alcohol syndrome. The centre is administered by the Greater Vancouver Fetal Alcohol Society, an organization that undertakes prevention activities and advocates on behalf of individuals and their families.

B.C. FAS Resource Society

Ms. Julianne Conry - Chair
P.O. Box 525
Maple Ridge, BC V2X 3P2

Services: The Society facilitates the development and dissemination of information and research, support and services for families, professionals and the broader community around prevention, intervention and treatment issues relating to FAS/FAE and other disabilities caused by alcohol and drug use during pregnancy.

Bulkley Valley FAS Prevention Committee

Ms. Cheryl Wickson
Box 2920
Smithers, BC V0J 2N0

Tel: (250) 847-8959 Fax: (250) 847-8974
Email: cherwick@hotmail.com

Services: This community-based Committee is involved in FAS awareness and prevention projects, advocacy, support, information provision and resource development.

Campbell River FAS/E Community Action Network

Ms. Mary Catherine Bellamy - Chairperson
Upper Island Central Coast Community Health Services Society
200 - 1100 Island Highway
Campbell River, BC V9W 8C6
Tel: (250) 286-0955 Fax: (250) 287-2822

Services: This is an informal multidisciplinary group of service providers that meet at regular intervals and work toward decreasing the occurrence of FAS/FAE in the community by developing effective and supportive services to families with substance abuse issues; educational support to children and teachers; effective services and programs for teens and young adults with FAS/FAE. This is done through a variety of projects, activities, educational events, and strengthening the work of the helping agencies in the community. A community action strategy for drug and alcohol abuse prevention is being developed.

Cowichan Valley FAS Action Team

Ms. Ro deBree
R.R. #3
3925 Vaux Road
Duncan, BC V9L 6S6
Tel: (250) 748-5115
Email: ro@islandnet.com

Services: The Action Team coordinates prevention and awareness activities within the community, advocates with and for people with Fetal Alcohol Syndrome and their families, and provides education for professionals and support for parents. They have recently developed "Finding Alternative Solutions," a mentorship program concentrating on in-services for groups of professionals who want to hear from young people with FAS. Publications available for purchase: "Jaycee," a book for families and children about a child with FAS ($7.00); "And Have Not Love," a book of poetry written by Leon's

Mom and "Your Victory; a Happy Child" written by Ro deBree. All are available through FAS Bookshelf.

Crabtree Corner (YWCA) FAS/NAS Prevention Program

Ms. Nola Harper - FAS Project Coordinator
101 East Cordova Street
Vancouver, BC V6A 1K7
Tel: (604) 689-2808 Fax: (604) 689-5463
Email: nharper@ywcavan.org
URL: ywcavan.org/families/index.html

Services: Crabtree is an emergency short-term daycare and family drop-in centre offering a variety of programs for women and children including education and training in the areas of FAS and NAS. The centre also provides advocacy, referral and support to women with children affected by FAS. Resource material is available to the community and outreach education programs are available to consumer groups.

Duncan SNAP/FAS Parent Support

Ms. Marjorie Wilson
P.O. Box 1217
Lake Cowichan, BC V0R 2G0
Tel: (250) 749-3546

Services: Ms. Wilson is available for information, support and advocacy for families and individuals living with FAS.

FAS Bookshelf Inc.

Ms. Peggy Lasser
438 - 6540 East Hastings Street
Burnaby, BC V5B 4Z5
Tel: (604) 942-2024 Fax: (604) 942-2041
Email: info@fasbookshelf.com
URL: www.fasbookshelf.com

Services: The FAS Bookshelf provides both an online and mail order service for resources on FAS. Ms. Lasser has written a Vancouver School Board published handbook for teachers *Challenges and Opportunities: A Handbook for Teachers of Students with Special Needs with a Focus on FAS.*

FAS/E Support Network of B.C.

13279 - 72nd Avenue
Surrey, BC V3W 2N5
Tel: (604) 507-6675 (1 866) 328-3273 Fax: (604) 507-6685
Email: info@fetalalcohol.com
URL: www.fetalalcohol.com

Services: The Network provides consultation, education and support services and undertakes research projects in the area of FAS. Consultation and support services are under contract to the province of BC, Ministry for Children and Families, and are offered free of cost to users. Training services are available on a fee-for-service basis. Publications available for purchase include a newsletter "About FASE" four times per year, a series of six age-appropriate FASNET screening tools, "A layman's guide to fetal alcohol syndrome and possible fetal alcohol effects," "Dear world: we have fetal alcohol syndrome: experiences of young adults," "FAS/E and education: the art of making a difference," "My name is Amanda and I have FAE" and "So your child has FAS/E: what you need to know." The Network is currently developing a Canada wide training manual entitled *FAS/E: A Manual for Community Caring.*

FAS In Action

c/o Upper Island/Central Coast Community Health Services Society
961 England Avenue
Courtenay, BC V9N 2N7
Tel: (250) 338-1711 Fax: (250) 338-9985

Services: FAS In Action is a non-profit society and includes various members from the community including parents, Public Health Nursing, Family Services, John Howard Society, Wachiay Native Friendship Centre, the Infant Development Program, family literacy, the school district and foster parents. Public education and awareness, distribution of information, referral and support with regard to FAS/E issues are some of the activities undertaken within the community. You can also contact Mr. Bernie Monaghan at (250) 890-2093 or Ms. Joanne Mawhinney at (250) 334-4788.

Fetal Alcohol Syndrome Community Development Project

Ms. Kim Lyster - Regional Manager
Pat Richardson, Regional Coordinator
Penticton, BC

Tel: Kim: (250) 492-5814; Pat: (250) 861-3952 Fax: Kim: (250) 492-7572; Pat: (250) 861-3903
Email: kplyster@vip.net; patrichardson@shaw.ca

Services: This project aims to network and sustain FAS community teams in Penticton, Kelowna, Vernon and Salmon Arm; provide outreach to on reserve and urban First Nations communities, identify and respond to issues and needs emerging from communities: training, diagnostic and treatment services; provide support to families, individuals with FAS and professionals; provide information and resources to the region; liaise with provincial and national FAS initiatives and coordinate and deliver training events.

FOCUS Employment Program

Ms. Linda Schmidt
College of New Caledonia
Box 5000
Burns Lake, BC V0J 1E0
Tel: (250) 692-1700 Fax: (250) 692-1750
Email: schmidt@cnc.bc.ca

Services: Focus Employment Program is a specialized program for adults affected by Fetal Alcohol Syndrome/partial Fetal Alcohol Syndrome who are interested in gaining employment. The program stresses employer and community education and awareness and utilizes alternative learning strategies designed specifically for adults with learning difficulties.

Kelowna FAS/FAE Community Resource Team

Mr. Randy James
309 - 1664 Richter Street
Kelowna, BC V1Y 8N3
Tel: (250) 860-5183 Fax: (250) 860-9146
Email: rjames@paralynx.com

Services: The mission of the FAS/FAE Community Resource Team is to reduce the incidence of FAS/FAE in the Central Okanagan and to ameliorate the personal, social and economic consequences for affected individuals and their families. Team membership includes representation from community agencies and individuals, provincial government ministries, family physicians, pediatricians, and funding partners with a focus on prevention and intervention.

Kelowna FAS/SNAP Support Group

Ms. Pat Richardson
Kelowna, BC
Tel: (250) 861-3934 Fax: (250) 861-3903
Email: patrichardson@shaw.com

Services: The group provides parenting information and support, coordinates a monthly support group, and accepts speaking engagements.

Mackenzie SNAP Group

Ms. Chris Primus - Manager
P.O. Box 1793
Mackenzie, BC V0J 2C0
Tel: (250) 997-3090
Email: cdprimus@uniserve.com

Services: This group provides support, assistance and information to parents, caregivers, teachers and others who care for or work with individuals affected by FAS.

Maple Ridge FAS/ADD Resource Centre

Ms. Beryl Trimble
12161 - 221st Street
Maple Ridge, BC V2X 5T2
Tel: (604) 463-6750 Fax: (604) 463-6750
Email: berylt@telus.net
URL: www3.telus.net/berylt

Services: This Group provides information and resource materials covering FAS/FAE/ADD/ ADHD with a particular interest in aiming to identify the needs of adults and seniors and advocate for appropriate resources and health support. An online FAS/FAE/ADD/ADHD Chat Room is now open which can be accessed from the website. Meetings take place every Thursday at 7 p.m. (Pacific Time).

Peace River Liard Early Intervention Program

Ms. Lynn Locher - Manager
10141 - 101 Avenue
Fort St. John, BC V1J 2B3
Tel: (250) 785-6021 Fax: (250) 785-4659
Email: llocher@pris.bc.ca

Services: Through a consortium of the Child Development Centre Society of Fort St. John & District, and the North Peace Community Resource Society, the group provides assessment and diagnostic clinics for children, pregnancy outreach and prevention programs and follow-up services for individuals diagnosed with FAS/FAE. Parent support and building community capacity programs are available in Fort Nelson, Chetwynd, Fort St. John and Dawson Creek.

Penticton FAS Support Group

Ms. Penny Poitras
or Jo-Anne Thompson
126 Braelyn Crescent
Penticton, BC V2A 6V3
Tel: Penny: (250) 493-4915; Jo-Anne: (250) 770-8295
Email: pennypoitras@hotmail.com; jothompson@telus.net

Services: This support group is for caregivers of children with FAS/FAE and meetings are held on a monthly basis.

Powell River Association for Community Living

Ms. Liz Kellough
201 - 4675 Marine Avenue
Powell River, BC V8A 2L2
Tel: (604) 485-6411 Fax: (604) 485-6419
Email: pracl@prcn.org

Services: The Association offers a variety of programs and activities related to prevention and support to individuals with FAS/FAE as follows: infant development consultation and weekly parent and child play groups, preschool program and child care and family support services, pediatric physiotherapy, summer recreation programs for children from 5 through 18 years of age, transition program for young adults, adult day programs and a resource library.

Provincial FAS/NAS Early Intervention Consultant

Ms. Janet Amos
The Aurora Centre, 5th Floor
4500 Oak Street
Vancouver, BC V6H 3N1
Tel: (604) 875-2017 Fax: (604) 875-2039

Services: The early intervention consultant works with health and social service providers towards the provision of improved early intervention approaches with women at risk and gathers and disseminates information on effective early intervention strategies and appropriate and accessible treatment for women using alcohol and other drugs during pregnancy.

Provincial FAS Prevention Consultant

Ms. Anne Fuller
Ministry for Children and Families
P.O. Box 9719, Station Provincial Government
Victoria, BC V8W 9S1
Tel: (250) 952-6024 Fax: (250) 953-4556
Email: anne.fuller@gems8.gov.bc.ca

Services: The prevention consultant is responsible for promoting and supporting a network of information and expertise on FAS/ADRDD prevention among programs and projects throughout the province, providing information and referral services for the public and professionals on how to access related resources, expertise and services and to provide technical support to groups and organizations initiating activities at the community level.

Sal'i'Shan Institute Society

Mr. Bill Mussell - Principal Educator/Manager
Ms. Marion Mussell, Administrator
P.O. Box 242
800 Wellington Avenue
Chilliwack, BC V2P 6J1
Tel: (604) 792-7300 Fax: (604) 792-5498
Email: salishan@dowco.com

Services: The Society provides education and training programs for community health workers and addiction counsellors who may work with fetal alcohol affected persons with a primary focus on prevention and intervention.

Salmon Arm FAS Committee

Ms. Penny Ogasawara
c/o SECA Infant Development Program
Salmon Arm, BC
Tel: (250) 832-4921 Fax: (250) 832-4591

Services: This community team focuses on FAS awareness, prevention and increasing knowledge and support for individuals with FAS and their families.

SNAP - Society of Special Needs Adoptive Parents

Mr. Brad Watson - Executive Director
205 - 409 Granville Street
Vancouver, BC V6C 1T2
Tel: (604) 687-3114; 1(800) 663-7627 (BC only)
Fax: (604) 687-3364
Email: snap@snap.bc.ca URL: www.snap.bc.ca

Services: The Society of Special Needs Adoptive Parents (SNAP) provides support, information and education services to families who have adopted children with special needs, and the professionals who work with those families throughout the province. SNAP offers support groups, a one-to-one contact resource parent network, education workshops, and conferences on adoption and special needs issues, particularly FAS. The Society operates a toll-free in B.C. telephone contact line and publishes a quarterly news magazine and other information materials (such as the recently revised book *Parenting Children Affected by Fetal Alcohol Syndrome: A Guide for Daily Living*). SNAP also maintains a Resource Lending Library with over 9000 items – books, periodicals, reports, audio and video tapes and even some games. SNAP is a provincially registered, non-profit society and a federally registered charity. Membership is open to anyone interested in special needs adoption issues.

Sunshine Coast Community Services Society

Ms. Vicki Dobbyn
P.O. Box 1069
Sechelt, BC V0N 3A0
Tel: (604) 885-5881 Fax: (604) 885-9493
Email: community_services@sunshine.net

Services: This Society provides family counselling or referral and support for children and families affected by FAS/FAE.

Task Group - FAS

Ms. Terri Smith
12640 Laity Street
Maple Ridge, BC V4R 2P2

Tel: (604) 466-8904

Email: terri@telus.net

Services: This group provides support to parents.

Terrace Child Development Centre

Ms. Margot Van Kleeck - Executive Director

2510 South Eby Street

Terrace, BC V8G 2X3

Tel: (250) 635-9388 Fax: (250) 638-0213

Email: tcdc@osg.net

Services: The Centre provides counselling, information sessions and weekly meetings for pregnant women at risk and provides assessment for individuals as well as therapy and support for pre- school children with FAS and their families.

Vernon and District Fetal Alcohol Syndrome Initiative

Mr. Barry Brazier

Vernon, BC

Tel: (250) 542-9290

Email: bbrazier@shaw.ca

Services: This FAS community team is made up of professionals and parents of children with FAS. The objectives of the team are to find opportunities to increase community awareness about FAS prevention and best practice interventions for individuals with FAS and their families.

Manitoba

Brandon Inter Agency FAS/FAE Committee

Ms. Viola Fleury

510 Frederick Street

Brandon, MB R7A 6Z4

Tel: (204) 729-3845 Fax: (204) 729-3844

Email: vfleury@afm.mb.ca

Services: The Brandon Inter Agency FAS/FAE Committee is organized exclusively for the purposes of preventing Fetal Alcohol Syndrome and Fetal Alcohol Effects, and of establishing effective community resources in support of caregivers/parents and those affected.

Child Health and FAS Consultant

Ms. Dawn Ridd
Child Health Unit, Manitoba Health
2097 - 300 Carlton Street
Winnipeg, MB R3B 3M9
Tel: (204) 788-6667 Fax: (204) 948-2366
Email: dridd@gov.mb.ca

Services: Child Health provides leadership and coordination to the development of policies and programs respecting the health of infants, children and youth in Manitoba. Child Health works collaboratively with other government departments and community organizations to promote population health strategies to improve health outcomes for children, youth and families. Initiatives that are undertaken emphasize the importance of supporting overburdened families of young children, preventing prenatal and childhood intentional and unintentional injury, supporting early diagnosis and treatment initiatives, and developing/participating in partnerships to address issues such as Fetal Alcohol Syndrome prevention, improved community health care in schools, and Prenatal and Early Childhood Nutrition.

Clinic for Alcohol and Drug Exposed Children

Ms. Mary Cox Millar - Coordinator
Children's Hospital
CK-275, 840 Sherbrook Street
Winnipeg, MB R3A 1S1
Tel: (204) 787-1822; (204) 787-1828 Fax: (204) 787-1138
Email: sdion@hsc.mb.ca

Services: The Clinic provides multi-disciplinary assessment and diagnostic services, helps families link with appropriate resources in their community and develops strategies to increase knowledge and diagnostic capabilities in rural and isolated communities. Referrals are accepted for children up to the age of 18 years, where there has been pre-natal exposure to alcohol and/or drugs. Televideo diagnostic services are also available.

Coalition on Alcohol and Pregnancy

Mr. Dale Kendel - Chair
c/o Association for Community Living - Manitoba
210 - 500 Portage Avenue
Winnipeg, MB R3C 3X1

Tel: (204) 786-1607 Fax: (204) 789-9850
Email: aclmb@mb.sympatico.ca

Services: The Coalition is made up of a number of core committees whose members undertake FAS activities with respect to training, education, daycare, family, child welfare, justice, medical, adult services, rural development, research, media, and women's issues. Please contact the Coalition for a list of members and committees. An information resource centre is also available.

FAS Information Manitoba

Ms. Deborah Kacki
49 - 476 King Street
Winnipeg, MB R2W 3Z5
Tel: Toll Free: 1-866-877-0050

Services: The FAS Information Manitoba phone line provides information to Manitobans regarding alcohol related disabilities. The goals of the information line are: to offer accurate information on substance use during pregnancy; to provide families with information and strategies on parenting children/supporting individuals who have been prenatally exposed to alcohol; to offer an avenue for accessing community resources.

Fetal Alcohol Family Association of Manitoba Inc.

Ms. Kathy Jones - President
Leilana Buschau, Executive Director
210 - 500 Portage Avenue
Winnipeg, MB R3C 3X1
Tel: (204) 786-1847 Fax: (204) 789-9850
Email: fafa@mb.sympatico.ca
URL: www.fafam.ca

Services: The Fetal Alcohol Family Association of Manitoba Inc. provides advocacy, support and education to families caring for and professionals working with individuals who have been prenatally exposed to alcohol and/or drugs.

Flin Flon/Creighton FAS/FAE Committee

Ms. Janet Modler
Children's Special Services
50 Church Street

Flin Flon, MB R8A 1K5
Tel: (204) 687-1718 Fax: (204) 687-1708
Email: jmodler@gov.mb.ca

Services: This is a volunteer committee made up of parents and professionals interested in FAS issues. Activities include sponsoring training events for parents, teachers and foster parents. Members are available to provide prevention information to community groups or individuals. Children's Special Services provides support to families who have children with developmental and/or physical disabilities and who have children diagnosed with ARBD and have a concurrent developmental delay.

Frontier School Resource Program/Stop FAS Community Committee

Ms. Lia Braun - Special Services Consultant
Frontier School Division No. 48
General Delivery, Area V Office
Norway House, MB R0B 1B0
Tel: (204) 359-6711 Fax: (204) 359-6897
Email: lbraun@frontiersd.mb.ca

Services: Frontier S.D. has published "Making the Right Choices: A Grade 5-8 Fetal Alcohol Prevention Curriculum" which contains ready-to-use lesson plans. The Resource program staff are knowledgeable and experienced in working with alcohol-affected students and the teachers who work with these children. Frontier is a founding member of the Norway House Community Round Table Committee on FAS.

Interagency FAS/E Program

Ms. Deborah Kacki - Coordinator
49 - 476 King Street
Winnipeg, MB R2W 3Z5
Tel: (204) 582-8658 Fax: (204) 586-1874
Email: itafas@mb.sympatico.ca

Services: This program is for children aged 0 through 6, who have been diagnosed with an alcohol-related disability, or whose birth mothers have acknowledged prenatal exposure to harmful substances. It offers support and education services for the children and their caregivers at home, in daycare and within the school system.

Nor'West Mentor Program

Ms. Cathe Umlah - Coordinator
103 - 61 Tyndall Avenue
Winnipeg, MB R2X 2T4
Tel: (204) 632-8162 Fax: (204) 632-4666
Email: norwest@escape.ca

Services: This is an FAS/E prevention program working with high risk women in the community who are pregnant and drinking and/or using drugs.

The Pas Inter-Agency FAS/FAE Committee

Ms. Donna Janzen
Child and Family Services
Box 2550
The Pas, MB R9A 1M4
Tel: (204) 627-8225 Fax: (204) 623-5792
Email: djanzen@gov.mb.ca; janzend@mb.sympatico.ca

Services: This is a volunteer committee consisting of parents and professionals who are interested in enhancing services to FAS/FAE children and families in the community.

West Region Child and Family Services

Ms. Kathy Jones - Children with Special Needs Coordinator
704 - 167 Lombard Avenue
Winnipeg, MB R3V 0V3
Tel: (204) 957-0037; (204) 985-4050 Fax: (204) 985-4079

Services: West Region Child and Family Services is a First Nation Child Welfare agency that provides services to children and families on nine reserve communities in Western Manitoba. Through the FAS program, the agency provides consultation and support to families affected by FAS/E. Programs include school support, counselling to children and parents, consultation on the needs of affected children and presentations and workshops. The agency also co-publishes "Tough Kids and Substance Abuse," a program for youth with FAS who are at risk for using alcohol and/or other drugs, and runs a yearly gathering called Reclaiming Our Voices: A Gathering for Women Who Drank While They Were Pregnant, held each fall.

New Brunswick

The Union of New Brunswick Indians Training Institute

370 Wilsey Road
Fredericton, NB E3B 6E9
Tel: (506) 458-9444 Fax: (506) 458-2850
Email: unbiti@unbi.org

Services: Prevention and training/education workshops and information sessions on FAS/FAE can be delivered throughout the Maritimes. Resource materials may also be borrowed.

Newfoundland

Aboriginal Family Centre

Ms. Jenny Lyall
or Lois Roberts
P.O. Box 1949, Station B
38 Grenfell Street
Happy Valley - Labrador, NF A0P 1E0
Tel: (709) 896-4398/4399 Fax: (709) 896-4408
Email: afc@hvgb.net

Services: The FAS/FAE Steering Committee provides resource material within the Labrador region.

Labrador Inuit Health Commission Resource Centre

Ms. Winnie Healey - Resource Technician
P.O. Box 234
North West River, Labrador, NF A0P 1M0
Tel: (709) 497-8356 Fax: (709) 497-8311
Email: healeyw@hvgb.net

Services: The Centre provides information and resource materials for the region on FAS prevention and awareness.

Nova Scotia

FAS/FAE Support Network of Nova Scotia

Mr. Tom Coffey
30 Sherry Avenue
Kentville, NS B4N 1Z7

Tel: (902) 678-0281
Email: tom.coffey@ns.sympatico.ca

Services: This support network is for parents and caregivers of children with FAS/FAE and its aim is to help in advocating for services and interventions for families. Also contact: Chris Collins, 7 1/2 Levis Street, Halifax, NS B3R 1M2. Tel: (902) 479-1573.

Mi'kmaq First Nation Healing Society

Ms. Della Maguire - Executive Director
2209 Bishopville Road
Hantsport, NS B0P 1P0
Tel: (902) 684-0104
Email: della@ns.sympatico.ca

Services: The Society is a non-profit organization serving Aboriginal people in Atlantic Canada. The goal of the Society is to provide workshops to empower the aboriginal communities through education, training, support and healing regarding FAS/FAE and Residential School issues. The Society provides on-going training and educational sessions for communities and organizations across Canada. A training manual "Empowering Our Communities on FAS/FAE" is available at a cost of $22.50 (includes shipping and handling).

Program Consultant, Atlantic Region

Ms. Teresa Palliser
Population and Public Health Branch
18th Floor Maritime Centre
1802 - 1505 Barrington Street
Halifax, NS B3J 3Y6
Tel: (902) 426-7148 Fax: (902) 426-9689
Email: teresa_jeffery@hc-sc.gc.ca

Services: Please contact for information about FAS/FAE programs and activities in the Atlantic Region, as well as for Aboriginal Head Start Programs in the Atlantic Region.

Reproductive Health

Ms. Lona Hegeman - Consultant
Department of Health and Social Services
P.O. Box 1320, CST-7
Yellowknife, NT X1A 2L9
Tel: (867) 873-7051; 1-800-661-0782 (toll free in NT)
Fax: (867) 873-0202
Email: lona_hegeman@gov.nt.ca

Services: The consultant supports regional health boards and territorial organizations in their FAS prevention and awareness initiatives. The consultant implements and promotes the departmental FAS prevention and awareness initiatives and represents the NWT on the Prairie Northern Pacific FAS Partnership comprised of Manitoba, Saskatchewan, Alberta, BC, Yukon, Nunavut and the NWT.

Yellowknife Association for Community Living

Ms. Doreen Baptiste - Coordinator
Living and Learning with FAS Project
P.O. Box 981
Yellowknife, NT X1A 2N7
Tel: (867) 873-9069 Fax: (867) 669-7826
Email: yaclfas@ssimicro.com

Services: The Living and Learning with FAS project, funded by Health Canada, works from a community development perspective offering FAS education, awareness and family support services. Project activities are guided by an FAS Community Team made up of a variety of community agencies, families, health professionals and government representatives.

Nunavut

Baffin Fetal Alcohol Network

Ms. Janice Beddard
P.O. Box 143
Iqaluit, NU X0A 0H0
Tel: (867) 979-0741 Fax: (867) 979-5994
Email: JBeddard@qikiqtani.edu.nu.ca

Services: This is a network of community volunteers working in the area of prevention and education. Resource materials (including videos and print material in Inuktitut) are available and presentations to groups or organizations can be arranged.

Ontario

Amethyst Women's Addiction Centre

Ms. Carol Wu - Coordinator
488 Wilbrod Street
Ottawa, ON K1N 6M8
Tel: (613) 563-0363 Fax: (613) 565-2175
Email: amethyst@eisa.com amedirector@eisa.com
URL: ww.amethyst-ottawa.org

Services: Amethyst accommodates women who are pregnant by ensuring they can enter into the treatment program well before their due date. Amethyst offers support to women with children with FAS/FAE, provides a parenting group and children's program and offers referrals as necessary.

Breaking the Cycle

Ms. Margaret Leslie - Program Manager
761 Queen Street West, Suite 107
Toronto, ON M6J 1G1
Tel: (416) 364-7373, ext. 204 Fax: (416) 364- 8008
Email: mleslie@mothercraft.org
URL: www.breakingthecycle.ca

Services: Breaking the Cycle is a prevention and early intervention project designed to reduce risk and enhance the development of sub-stance-exposed children (prenatal-6 yrs) by addressing maternal addiction problems and the mother-child relationship in a single-access, community-based model. Through the efforts of 6 partner agencies (Mothercraft, The Jean Tweed Centre, Children's Aid Society of Toronto, Catholic Children's Aid Society, Hospital for Sick Children and Toronto Department of Public Health), the program offers integrated addiction counselling, parenting, health/medical, pregnancy outreach and child developmental services to women who are pregnant and/or have young children, and have substance use problems. Breaking the Cycle is funded by Health Canada's CAPC and CPNP programs.

FASAT (Ontario)

Ms. Chris Margetson - Executive Director
c/o Homewood Health Center, CADS
100 - 49 Emma Street
Guelph, ON N1E 6X1
Tel: (519) 822-2476 Fax: (519) 822-4895
Email: fasat@golden.net
URL: home.golden.net/~fasat

Services: This organization has been developed in order to meet the needs of children across Ontario with FAS/FAE by providing training for the professionals and parents who work with and care for them, by advocating and supporting families and by being involved in activities related to prevention.

FASlink (Fetal Alcohol Spectrum Disorders Information, Support & Communications Link)

Mr. Bruce Ritchie - Moderator
2445 Old Lakeshore Road
Bright's Grove, ON N0N 1C0
Tel: (519) 869-8026 Fax: (519) 869-8026
Email: fas@acbr.com
URL: www.acbr.com/fas

Services: FASlink is a moderated email discussion group that provides support and information for individuals, families and professionals who are working with and caring for those affected by prenatal alcohol exposure. FASlink serves more than 200 000 visitors to its website annually. The FASlink Archives contain more than 70 000 letters and articles on FAS issues. FASlink's online discussion forum is the primary Canadian FAS communications network and includes members worldwide. FASlink publishes the FASlink CDROM and FAS InfoDisk (for download from the website). To join the list serv, send an email message to: majordomo@listserv.rivernet.net and, leaving the subject line blank, type – subscribe faslink – in the body of the message.

FASworld Toronto

Ms. Mary Cunningham - President
Brian Philcox, Executive Director
1509 Danforth Avenue

Toronto, ON M4J 5C3
Tel: (416) 465-7766 Fax: (416) 465-8890
Email: fasworldcanada@home.ca
URL: www.fasworld.com

Services: Originally founded as Fetal Alcohol Support Network (Metropolitan Toronto and Peel), the group has changed its name in order to become the first chapter of FASworld Canada. The group meets on the second Saturday of the month at St. Michael's Hospital in Toronto in order to support families with members struggling with FASD. Membership is open to parents, care givers, professionals and others interested in FASD prevention. Call Brian for further information.

Fetal Alcohol Information Support Network

Ms. Theone Collins
P.O. Box 20022
150 Churchill Blvd.
Sault Ste. Marie, ON P6A 6W3
Tel: (705) 946-0638 Fax: (705) 946-3004
Email: the1collins.fassm@sympatico.ca
URL: www.soonet.ca/faisn

Services: The Network undertakes activities to help prevent alcohol related birth defects and provides support and information to those affected.

Fetal Alcohol Support and Information Centre

Mr. & Mrs. Bill & Joan Smith
6790 Charlie Brooks Court
Windsor, ON N8T 3L6
Tel: (519) 948-8599 Fax: (519) 948-3527
Email: faswindsor@cogeco.ca

Services: The Centre provides a support group and information resources for parents and caregivers of children with FAS and will participate as speakers or presenters at seminars and workshops.

Fetal Alcohol Support and Information Network (F.A.S.I.N.)

Mr. & Mrs. Dave and Margie Fulton
P.O. Box 100
Murillo, ON P0T 2G0

Tel: (807) 935-3168 Fax: (807) 935-2198
Email: fulton@northroute.net

Services: FASIN works towards creating more awareness in the community about FAS/FAE, assists and supports families and individuals and responds to requests for information. Regularly scheduled meetings are held where people have the opportunity to gain an understanding of FAS/E, as well as problem solve around specific issues. Meetings with individuals, families or interested professionals are also arranged as needed. Occasional special family activities are organized. Displays, presentations, and workshops on a variety of topics are arranged as needed.

Fetal Alcohol Syndrome Association of Ottawa (FASAO)

Ms. Elspeth Ross
Box 915
Rockland, ON K4K 1L5
Tel: (613) 737-1122; (613) 446-4144 Fax: (613) 446-4144
Email: rosse@freenet.carleton.ca

Services: FASAO provides support for families, and information and education for families and professionals on the effects of alcohol on people of all ages, and importance of prevention. Monthly meetings are held from October to June at the Children's Hospital of Eastern Ontario (CHEO). Please contact Elspeth Ross for further details.

Fetal Alcohol Syndrome Treatment and Education Centre Inc.

Ms. Jill Dockrill
194 Foster Avenue
Belleville, ON K8N 3P9
Tel: (613) 968-8129 Fax: (613) 968-5263
Email: jillfastec@netscape.net

Services: A registered nonprofit organization whose mandate is awareness and prevention of FAS as well as advocating for programs and services for individuals affected by prenatal alcohol exposure. We are currently working towards establishing a Residential FAS Treatment and Education Centre.

Healthy Generations Family Support Program

Ms. Judy Kay
Sioux Lookout & Hudson Association for Community Living

Box 1258
Sioux Lookout, ON P8T 1B8
Tel: (807) 737-4600 Fax: (807) 737-3833
Email: healthy@slhacl.on.ca

Services: The program provides support for families raising children exposed to alcohol or drugs prenatally, or children with FAS and related conditions.

Kenora and area FAS/FAE Committee

Ms. Patti Dryden Holmstrom
c/o Addiction Services Kenora Youth Program Lake of the Woods District Hospital
12 Main Street South
Kenora, ON P9N 1S7
Tel: (807) 468-6770 Fax: (807) 468-6093
Email: pdryden@voyageur.ca

Services: The Committee undertakes activities related to prevention and community awareness.

Native Child and Family Services of Toronto

201 - 464 Yonge Street
Toronto, ON M4Y 1W9
Tel: (416) 969-8510 Fax: (416) 969-9251

Services: The following programs are available: Youth with FAS Support Group offers traditional and contemporary approaches to support aboriginal youth with FASD between the ages of 16-24; Children with FASD five day summer camp offers a safe and structured environment for children between the ages of 8 - 12, providing respite for caregivers; Parents with FASD Support Group is offered once a week and provides ongoing support for parents living with FAS (diagnosed or undiagnosed); Parenting Children with FASD is a ten-week session that looks at education, behavioral and environmental techniques for caregivers and parents.

Ontario Federation of Indian Friendship Centres

Ms. Kim Meawasige - FAS/FAE Policy Analyst
219 Front Street East
Toronto, ON M5A 1E8

Tel: (416) 956-7575 Fax: (416) 956-7577
Email: kmeawasige@ofifc.org

Services: This program will assist with FAS/FAE resources available to urban Aboriginal people in Ontario. It offers both a traditional and contemporary approach to FAS, on-site training and consultations as well as intervention, prevention and programming including community development regarding FAS/FAE.

Sarnia/Lambton FAS/FAE Support Group

Ms. Deborah Dunn
388 Confederation Street
Sarnia, ON N7T 2A8
Tel: (519) 336-1576 Fax: (519) 336-7150
Email: ddunn40@rivernet.net
URL: www.rivernet.net/~fas

Services: The purpose of this group is to support, educate and inform. A poster is available for purchase entitled "Give your baby the best possible start in life."

South West Regional Fetal Alcohol Parent Advisory Group

Mrs. Susan Kampers
R.R. #3
23141 Thames Road
Appin, ON N0L 1A0
Tel: (519) 289-0155 Fax: (519) 289-0635
Email: susan.kampers@sympatico.ca

Services: This group provides support and education to families with children diagnosed with FAS and is involved in public speaking within the community.

Spring Cottage

Ms. Su Knorr - Executive Director
P.O. Box 247
Manotick, ON K4M 1A3
Tel: (613) 692-8254
Email: knorr@sprint.ca; spring_cottage@hotmail.com

Services: Spring Cottage provides a three-tiered intervention/prevention program, designed to promote health, prevent alcohol and drug use during pregnancy and break the cycle of addiction and the negative impact that it may have on future pregnancies. The primary prevention program will be done on an outreach basis with an emphasis on health promotion; the secondary program will be in partnership with an addictions program with intervention undertaken at the onset of pregnancy and the tertiary program will be implemented at Spring Cottage Recovery Home.

Waterloo FAS Support Group

Ms. Bonnie May
Regional Municipality of Waterloo Infant Development Program
P.O. Box 1612
99 Regina St. South, 5th Floor
Waterloo, ON N2J 4G6
Tel: (519) 883-2223 Fax: (519) 883-8102

Services: This is a support group for parents raising children suspected of prenatal alcohol exposure. Requests for informtion and for participation in workshops are responded to.

Prince Edward Island

Health and Social Services

P.O. Box 2000
Charlottetown, PE C1A 7N8
Tel: (902) 368-4273 Fax: (902) 368-6229
Email: dhoakes@ihis.org

Services: Addictions Services responds to requests for educational presentations regarding FAS/FAE issues and has produced three pamphlets for pregnant women: "What you should know about drugs," "What you should know about alcohol" and "What you should know about over the counter drugs."

PEI Reproductive Care Program

Ms. Diane Boswall - Coordinator
P.O. Box 2000
11 Kent Street
Charlottetown, PE C1A 7N8
Tel: (902) 368-4952 Fax: (902) 368-7537
Email: repcare@auracom.com

Services: This Program is involved in the prevention of FAS through the promotion of a comprehensive psychosocial assessment by physicians of all pregnant women. Assessment for alcohol use and abuse is one component of this assessment. Intervention and referral during the pregnancy is encouraged.

Québec

SAFERA (Syndrome d'Alcoolisation Foetale et Effets Reliés à l'Alcool)

Mme Louise Loubier-Morin - Présidente
845, chemin du Bord de l'eau
St-Henri, QC G0R 3E0
Tel: (418) 882-2488 Fax: (418) 882-2488
Email: info@safera.qc.ca
URL: www.safera.qc.ca

Services: SAFERA est un organisme canadien oeuvrant en français dont la mission est la prévention, l'information et la formation sur les effets de l'exposition prénatale à l'alcool, le SAF/EAF, et accessoirement sur les effets de l'exposition aux solvants et autres drogues.

Saskatchewan

Battlefords Family Health Centre

Ms. Charlotte Hamilton - Program Coordinator
Child Development Services
1192 - 101st Street, Room 103
North Battleford, SK S9A 0Z6
Tel: (306) 937-6840 Fax: (306) 445-4887
Email: chamilton@sk.sympatico.ca

Services: Women who are at risk for delivering a child with FAS/FAE are assessed and provided with supportive home based outreach services. Individual care plans are developed and resources are mobilized to meet their needs and to protect their unborn child.

Kinsmen Children's Centre

Alvin Buckwold Child Development Program
1319 Colony Street

Saskatoon, SK S7N 2Z1
Tel: (306) 655-1070 Fax: (306) 655-1449

Services: The Centre serves children's special health needs that may include physical and intellectual disabilites and/or genetic metabolic disorders. Services provided by a team include assessment, diagnosis, consultation, treatment and management of children and youth suspected of having Fetal Alcohol Syndrome (FAS), Partial FAS, Alcohol Related Neurodevelopmental Disorder (ARND) or Alcohol Related Birth Defects (ARBD). Periodic reviews of the child's development may also be done at 5 and 10 years. On site is a Family Resource Room which supports families by providing current information on disabilities as well as the services and programs available to help children with special needs and their families. A lending library of books and print resources is available.

Northern Interdepartmental Committee for the Prevention of FAS/FAE

Ms. Kyla McKenzie - Chairperson
Box 1379
La Ronge, SK S0J 1L0
Tel: (306) 425-5511 Fax: (306) 425-5335
Email: kmckenzie@cableronge.sk.ca

Services: This committee coordinates educational opportunities for professional/community/ family members on the issue of FAS and acts as an advisory committee for special community projects, networking and resource sharing.

Regina FAS/E Interagency Network

Ms. Anne Pinay - Co-chair
3510 - 5th Avenue
Regina, SK S4T 0M2
Tel: (306) 766-7540 Fax: (306) 766-7534

Services: This is a network of human service professionals and others from the community working to address issues and advocate for services for individuals affected by FAS/E and their families. You may also contact Tara Sylvester, Co-chair at (306) 780- 7572 or by email: sylvestertl@csc-scc.gc.ca.

Saskatchewan Clinical Teratology Program

Dr. Patricia M. Blakley
Department of Pediatrics, Royal University Hospital
103 Hospital Drive
Saskatoon, SK S7N 0W8
Tel: (306) 655-1096 Fax: (306) 655-1449
Email: blakleyp@sdh.sk.ca

Services: The Program provides pre-conception, prenatal and postnatal assessments in regard to drug exposure during pregnancy. A major focus of the Program is the diagnosis and management of children prenatally exposed to alcohol. The Program also provides continuing medical education on issues relating to teratogenesis.

Saskatchewan Fetal Alcohol Support Network, Inc.

Ms. Marion Tudor - President/Caregiver
Mr. Terry Hellquist, Treasurer/Caregiver
P.O. Box 9744
Saskatoon, SK S7K 7G8
Tel: (306) 975-0884 Fax: (306) 242-8007
Toll Free: 1-866-673-FASN (3276)
Email: fas.esupportnetwork@sasktel.net
Office Hours: 9:00am - 4:30pm Monday to Friday

Services: The Network is a parent group working to unite families and interested professionals who live and work with individuals affected by Fetal Alcohol Syndrome and Fetal Alcohol Effect. The goal of the Network is to promote peer support and the exchange of information within the province to ultimately provide the best environment possible for all persons with FAS/FAE. The Network publishes a newsletter: "Living With FAS/E" available with a $15.00 membership fee.

Saskatchewan Institute on Prevention of Handicaps

Ms. Lois Crossman - FAS Program Coordinator
Ms. Holly Graham, FAS Educator
1319 Colony Street
Saskatoon, SK S7N 2Z1
Tel: (306) 655-2512 Fax: (306) 655-2511
Email: skiph@sk.sympatico.ca
URL: www.PreventionInstitute.sk.ca

Services: The Prevention Institute is a provincial nonprofit organization working to raise awareness of prevention measures to reduce the incidence of handicapping conditions in children. The Prevention Institute has developed and promoted FAS prevention awareness and education information through conferences, workshops and presentations as well as through the distribution of resources such as FAS Resource Kits, audiovisual materials and print information. The Institute administers a provincial FAS/FAE prevention program and coordinates activities of the Saskatchewan FAS Coordinating Committee in order to maximize the efforts of professionals, family and community organizations.

Saskatoon Association for Community Living

Ms. Jeanne Remenda - Executive Director
102 - 135 Robin Crescent
Saskatoon, SK S7L 6M3
Tel: (306) 652-9111 Fax: (306) 652-9112
Email: sacl@sk.sympatico.ca

Services: SACL advocates for services in the community on behalf of families who have a family member diagnosed with FAS/FAE.

Shadow Above FAS/FAE Support Group

Ms. Debra MacNutt - Group Organizer
105B - 378 Parkview Road
Yorkton, SK S3N 3A9
Tel: (306) 783-9609
Email: shadowabove@accesscomm.ca

Services: This support group which has started recently is for caregivers, family, friends or people with FAS/FAE in and around the Yorkton area.

Yukon

Alcohol and Drug Secretariat

Ms. Jocyline Gauthier - Prevention Consultant - FAS/E Initiatives
Yukon Health and Social Services
6118 - 6th Avenue
Whitehorse, YT Y1A 1M9
Tel: (867) 667-5780 Fax: (867) 667-8471
Email: jocyline.gauthier@gov.yk.ca

Services: Please contact for information on the FAS Working Group, Alcohol and Drug Services' FAS Prevention Initiative, the FAS prevention prenatal kit "Alcohol and the Unborn Baby" or FAS prevention education in the Yukon.

Fetal Alcohol Syndrome Society of Yukon (FASSY)

Ms. Judy Pakozdy - Executive Director
Box 31396
Whitehorse, YT Y1A 6K8
Tel: (867) 393-4948 Fax: (867) 393-4950
Email: fascap@yknet.yk.ca

Services: The Society's mandate is to make a difference for people with FAS and their families and has developed and cofacilitated workshops related to prevention, intervention and living with FAS. The Society also assists communities in developing sustainable community activities which support families as well as the community groups to work successfully with people with FAS and to prevent more affected babies from being born. A poster is available entitled "The Many Faces of Fetal Alcohol Syndrome" and a pamphlet, "How to Take Care of Your Baby Before Birth."

Options for Independence

Ms. Elaine Seier - Project Manager
c/o 201 - 4050 4th Avenue
Whitehorse, YT Y1A 1H2
Tel: (867) 633-4164 Fax: (867) 667-4337
Email: yaclwhse@yknet.yk.ca

Services: This is a three year pilot project (which began in 1999) that provides secure housing for adults with FAS/FAE.

Youth of Today Society

Ms. Victoria Durrant - Executive Director
Blue Feather Youth Drop-in and Resource Centre
2157 - 2nd Avenue
Whitehorse, YT Y1A 1C6
Tel: (867) 633-9687
Email: victoria_durrant@hotmail.com

Services: The Youth of Today Society (YOTS) is a non-profit, charitable society with special attention given towards addressing the needs of young people ages 14-22 whose lives have been affected by FAS/FAE. YOTS provides ongoing support and direction with special attention given towards prevention, provides a facility set up as a home with a kitchen and a feeding program, serving meals for up to 20 youth. As well, the program involves art, music and counselling on life and job skills development. It is a drop-in environment where youth and community partners work together to support each other.

Yukon Association for Community Living

Ms. Vicki Wilson
P.O. Box 31478
Whitehorse, YT Y1A 6K8
Tel: (867) 667-4606 Fax: (867) 668-8169
Email: yaclwhse@yknet.yk.ca

Services: The Association maintains an information centre and advocates on behalf of individuals with FAS.

Index

fetal development (effect of toxic substances), 28, 33

First Steps program, 73-82, 85, 89, 90

foster parents/homes, 7, 47, 74, 93, 95, 99, 100, 105, 107

generalize (inability to), 31, 37, 40

glamorizing alcohol, 8

harm reduction, 9, 19, 71, 72

history of FASD, 25

home visitation/support, 72, 76, 79, 83, 84, 96

identification cards for FASD, 58, 59

ignorance of pregnancy, 34

impulsiveness, 31, 45, 47, 48, 57, 65, 67, 104, 109

incidence of FASD, 33, 78

intelligence/IQ, 31, 104, 105

Joining Forces, 98-100

judges, 43, 50, 53, 54, 55, 56, 57, 58, 63, 64, 65, 68, 86, 87

law librarians, 50, 57, 58

lawyers, 43, 57, 63, 64, 65, 66, 68, 77

learning disabilities, 12, 13, 37, 57, 88, 94, 107

legal aid, 49, 50, 54

LHI (Life History Interview), 60

memory problems, 31, 37, 46, 65, 94, 103, 104

mental fitness to stand trial, 47, 57, 64, 67

mental retardation, 29, 34

money (difficulty handling), 37, 57

multi-barrier individuals, 9, 10, 12, 13, 16, 19, 79, 80, 84, 85

"normal" appearance, 31, 45, 105

P-CAP (Parent-Child Assistance Program), 21, 71-73, 76

parenting courses, 93

police, 21, 42, 50, 51, 52, 53, 58, 59, 60, 63, 65, 68

poverty (1. see socio-economic status).

poverty (2. easy access for research), 16, 24, 34

pre-natal care, 34, 35

primary disabilities, 25, 26, 27, 28, 29, 30, 37, 107

prison/detention centres/correctional institutions, 12, 29, 46, 49, 63, 68, 69, 70

probation officers, 50, 55, 63, 64, 65, 66, 68, 77, 82

punishment (for crimes), 45, 55

rehabilitation, 47, 56, 61, 77, 78, 83

repetition (of behavior), 40, 61, 62, 65

safe amounts of alcohol during pregnancy, 7, 34

secondary disabilities, 7, 29, 31, 37, 40, 45, 47, 48, 60, 82, 88, 89, 90, 103, 105, 107

sex trade workers/prostitution, 15, 19, 40, 74

sexual behavior (inappropriate), 37, 109

social programs, 9, 71-91

social services, 7, 16, 48, 60, 65, 71, 72

social workers, 11, 49, 50, 57, 77, 80, 98, 100, 102

socio-economic status, 8, 10, 13, 16, 19, 20, 24, 34, 35, 43

Step by Step program, 82-87

time (poor concept of), 37, 38, 57, 63

Triumf Project, 60

victimization (risk of), 37, 61

Young Offenders Act, 19

Greening Your Pet Care

Darcy Matheson

Self-Counsel Press
(a division of)
International Self-Counsel Press Ltd.
USA   Canada

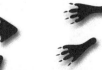
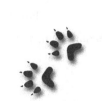
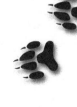

Self-Counsel Press acknowledges the financial support of the Government of Canada through the Canada Book Fund for our publishing activities.

Printed in Canada.

First edition: 2016

Library and Archives Canada Cataloguing in Publication

Matheson, Darcy, author
   Greening your pet care / Darcy Matheson.

ISBN 978-1-77040-261-4 (paperback)

   1. Pets—Environmental aspects. 2. Sustainable living. I. Title.

SF413.M32 2016   636.088'7   C2016-901571-8

Self-Counsel Press
(a division of)
International Self-Counsel Press Ltd.

Bellingham, WA   North Vancouver, BC
USA   Canada

Contents

Notice to Readers

Every effort is made to keep this publication as current as possible. However, the author, the publisher, and the vendor of this book make no representations or warranties regarding the outcome or the use to which the information in this book is put and are not assuming any liability for any claims, losses, or damages arising out of the use of this book. The reader should not rely on the author or the publisher of this book for any professional advice. Please be sure that you have the most recent edition.

Website links often expire or web pages move; at the time of this book's publication the links were current.

Dedication

Greening Your Pet Care is dedicated to the millions of fantastic companion animals that end up in shelters each year through no fault of their own — and those who have dedicated their lives to saving them. May your kindness result in empty cages.

To my long-suffering husband: Thank you for your love and patience, as always.

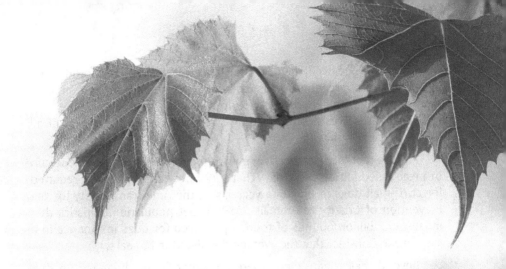

Introduction

Our population and our use of the finite resources of planet Earth are growing exponentially, along with our technical ability to change the environment for good or ill.

— Stephen Hawking

They're small, they're adorable, but few of us realize the enormous impact our companion animals have on the environment.

In their 2009 guide to sustainable living, authors Brenda and Robert Vale found that a medium-sized dog has a carbon footprint of 2.1 acres, roughly twice the 1 acre for a gas-guzzling sports utility vehicle driven 10,000 kilometers (6,214 miles) a year.[1] It's not just dogs that are contributing to pollution. The couple found that cats occupy the same footprint as a small Volkswagen, while two hamsters equal the same emissions as a plasma-screen television.

By their very nature, many family pets are carnivores, and it's that meat-eating diet that contributes to their substantial carbon footprint. Producing the grain and meat for pet food consumes a vast amount of

---

1 *Time to Eat the Dog: The Real Guide to Sustainable Living*, Brenda and Robert Vale.

resources — specifically land, energy, and water. That meat production belches harmful greenhouse gas emissions into the atmosphere in staggering amounts. The Food and Agriculture Organization of the United Nations estimates livestock production is responsible for 18 percent of all CO_2 emissions worldwide.[2]

Putting that into perspective, my 15-pound terriers each eat one cup of meat-based kibble every day. That's 730 pounds of pet food required for two small dogs in only one year. Using the American Society for the Prevention of Cruelty to Animals' (ASPCA) pet population statistics that means 29.2-billion pounds of food is produced for dogs in America in a single year. Consider that the average dog lives for 12 years.

Beyond their meaty diets, there are other factors bumping up that carbon "paw print." Animal waste and the plastic bags used to throw it away contribute to millions of tonnes of waste in municipal landfills each year, and pollute rivers and streams used for human drinking water. In my hometown alone, an estimated 97,000 tonnes of dog waste is disposed of in Metro Vancouver regional parks each year.

There's also all the bedding, clothes, toys, and supplies we lavish on our pets. Spending for pet products reached an all-time high of $60.5-billion in the US in 2015.[3] We're shelling out big bucks for many products that are plastic, bad for the planet, and not necessary to enhance and enrich the life and well-being of our pets.

The carbon footprint of our family pets is poised to grow exponentially in coming years. The number of household pets has more than doubled in the US since the 1970s, says the Humane Society, and tens of millions of North Americans now share their homes — and lives — with animals.[4] Fifty-seven-percent of Canadian households[5] and 65 percent of American households are now pet guardians.[6]

It's estimated there are up to 86 million dogs and 103 million cats owned in North America, and millions of rabbits, reptiles, snakes, turtles, hamsters, guinea pigs, and other small animals. More than 105-million fresh and saltwater fish are kept in home aquariums.[7]

Unlike previous generations where dogs were relegated to the backyard, it's now much more likely to see the family Fido in its master's bed

2 "Livestock's Long Shadow: Environmental Issues and Options," Food and Agriculture Organization of the United Nations, accessed January 2016. ftp.fao.org/docrep/fao/010/a0701e/a0701e00.pdf
3 "Pet Industry Spending at All-time High," The American Pet Products Association (APPA), accessed January 2016. media.americanpetproducts.org/press.php?include=145554
4 "Animal Sheltering Trends in the US," The Humane Society of the United States, accessed January 2016. humanesociety.org/animal_community/resources/timelines/animal_sheltering_trends.html
5 "Consumer Corner: Canadian Pet Market Outlook, 2014," Alberta Agriculture and Forestry, accessed January 2016. www1.agric.gov.ab.ca/$department/deptdocs.nsf/all/sis14914
6 "US Pet Industry Spending Figures & Future Outlook," American Pet Products Association (APPA), accessed January 2016. americanpetproducts.org/press_industrytrends.asp
7 Statistics compiled from "Consumer Corner: Canadian Pet Market Outlook, 2014," Alberta Agriculture and Forestry www1.agric.gov.ab.ca/$department/deptdocs.nsf/all/sis14914 and "Pet Statistics," American Society for the Prevention of Cruelty to Animals (ASPCA) aspca.org/about-us/faq/pet-statistics. Accessed January 2016.

than in a wooden doghouse. The vast majority of pet owners surveyed in 2014 (86 percent of dog owners and 89 percent of cat owners) said they considered their pets to be a part of their family.[8]

There are good reasons they are called companion animals. Pets provide friendship, lower our stress levels, act as emotional support, and have huge positive effects on our mental well-being, fitness, and happiness. So while we as human beings strive to make positive eco-friendly choices in our daily lives to reduce our own carbon footprint, it makes perfect sense that we extend those efforts to our family's smallest members.

This book will give you tips and strategies to become an eco-conscious pet owner, from the food and treats you buy to veterinarian care and the products you use in your home and garden. Each chapter provides simple everyday hints and actions that will lower your pets' carbon footprint for the sake of their health and well-being — and the future of our planet.

---

8   "Consumer Corner: Canadian Pet Market Outlook, 2014," Alberta Agriculture and Forestry, accessed January 2016. www1.agric.gov.ab.ca/$department/deptdocs.nsf/all/sis14914

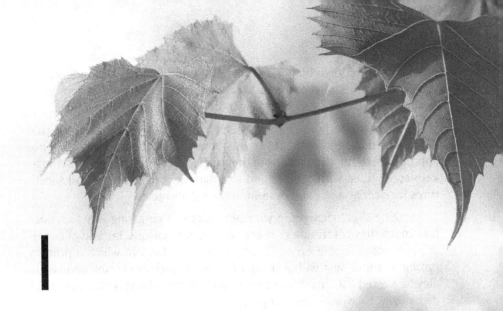

Ten Simple Steps to Going Green

No matter if your household pet is a four-ounce gerbil or a 140-pound Great Dane, there are simple things we can do make the lives of our companion animals less wasteful and harmful to our environment.

This chapter includes ten simple everyday steps you can take to make your pet ownership more eco-friendly.

1. Step 1: Avoid beef

Compared to any other animal, the production of beef has the most harmful effects on our planet. In a 2012 United Nations report on how meat production contributes to greenhouse gas emissions, factory-farm livestock production was identified as one of the top three most significant contributors to the world's current environmental problems, and a significant contributor to climate change.[1] Because of their feeding requirements, methane

---

1   UNEP Global Environmental Alert Service (GEAS), United Nations Environmental Programme, accessed January 2016. unep.org/pdf/unep-geas_oct_2012.pdf

production, and large body size, beef has a much larger carbon footprint than other forms of protein such as pork, chicken, turkey, sheep, goat, lamb, and rabbit, and exponentially more than grains and vegetables.

Because some household pets, such as cats, are "obligate" or true carnivores that require meat for their nutritional requirements, it's not appropriate to remove meat from their diets. However, the consumer marketplace is filled with choices and alternatives so it's easy to find substitutes for beef as a primary protein in their daily meals.

Making slight changes in your pets' diet will go a long way to reduce how much they contribute to greenhouse gas emissions. Instead of choosing beef-based kibble or wet food, switch to a food in which a primary protein is something with a smaller footprint, such as chicken or sustainably harvested fish. Just make sure to incorporate changes into your pet's diet slowly, to avoid stomach upset.

You can take it one step further by supplementing meals with foods that have a significantly smaller environmental footprint, such as pet-friendly non-animal proteins (e.g., legumes, cereals, grains, fruits, and vegetables). The same goes for treats: Look for grain, cereal, or fish-based treats instead of those sourced with beef.

With more than one-third of all spending on pets falling into the food category — an estimated $23-billion for 2015 alone, according to the American Pet Products Association — your individual choice can add up to a big difference. If more pet owners turn their back on beef-based pet food, less manufacturers will produce it because there will be less demand.

If you are ethically opposed to feeding your pet meat, there are quite a few options. Chapter 5 (dog care) discusses the matter of canines going vegetarian, and vegan food options. You can also opt for pets that don't require meat in their diet at all. Rabbits, for instance, are herbivores and not only are they vegetarian, but they'll happily gobble up any veggie trimmings and leftovers you have, — making them very eco-friendly companions.

2. Step 2: Reduce Your Transportation Footprint

Vehicle travel is one of the worst carbon emitters in most people's lives, but few of us think about how transportation pollution factors into the pet world.

It starts with where your animal comes from. Pets that come from large-scale commercial breeding facilities are often transported long distances by road and air to reach pet stores. Many wild-caught tropical fish are shipped from overseas. You can eliminate this carbon footprint by adopting from a shelter or rescue, or a reputable breeder in your area.

Next comes where you go for veterinary care and pet supplies. Look for a veterinarian close to your home — and seek pet food and products produced locally. If you are driving to the pet store to buy food, combine it with a trip to run errands so you're burning less fossil fuel.

3. Step 3: Don't Let Your Pet Run Wild

Letting your pet run wild has devastating effects on the environment and delivers a staggering blow to the natural world.

Believe it or not, the number one killer of birds in North America is cats. Far from flying under the radar, domestic and feral cats in Canada kill an estimated 196 million birds annually, which equates to 73 percent of total overall bird deaths. These killer kitties are responsible for more bird deaths than flying into power lines, houses, windows, or ingesting pesticides combined, according to a 2013 study by Avian Conservation & Ecology.[2]

Those figures are a drop in the bucket compared to the US, where a 2013 study in Nature Communications estimated that domestic cats are responsible for the death of 1.3 to 4 billion birds and 6.3 to 22.3 billion mammals annually.[3] After publishing the sobering figures, study authors identified cats as the "single greatest source of anthropogenic mortality for US birds and mammals" and called for policy intervention and conservation practices to reduce the death toll on the avian population.

Researchers on both sides of the border blamed "free-range" cats for the deaths, saying domestic cats permitted to roam outside unattended hunted without restraint — and were darned good at it. By nature, cats love hunting, especially at dusk and dawn. To reduce negative wildlife interactions, keep your cats indoors at all times. If your cats live primarily outdoors, try to keep them inside during those prime hunting periods.

Dogs are also notorious for terrorizing the natural terrain. Dogs that are allowed to be off-leash in sensitive ecological areas and beaches will often chase birds and other wildlife. Curious, clumsy canines are also a danger to nesting animals, not to mention growing plants and trees. Minimize damage by keeping your dog on a leash in these areas.

The biggest environmental damage from unsupervised and off-leash dogs comes from the "presents" they leave behind. Dog poop that isn't picked up by owners creates a risk to human health when it washes into and pollutes public waterways that are used for drinking water or recreation. In the 1990s, the US Environmental Protection Agency (EPA) classified pet waste as being just as toxic to the environment as chemical spills and oil.

---

2 "Estimated Number of Birds Killed by House Cats (*Felis catus*) in Canada," Avian Conservation & Ecology, accessed January 2016. ace-eco.org/vol8/iss2/art3/
3 "The Impact of Free-Ranging Domestic Cats on Wildlife of the United States," Scott R. Loss, Tom Will, and Peter P. Marra, Nature Communications, accessed January 2016. nature.com/ncomms/journal/v4/n1/full/ncomms2380.html

The EPA says the pathogens in dog and cat waste can cause a host of health concerns for humans if it ends up in their drinking water, including gastrointestinal illnesses, diarrhea, skin sores, and chest pain. Because the waste is nitrogen rich, it also depletes oxygen from the water, which harms fish and other water wildlife.

For rabbits and pocket-pet guardians, the bigger danger of having free-roaming pets is that they can become prey for other animals. Hawks, raccoons, cats, and dogs, can hunt domestic rabbits and small animals if they are left unattended outside.

Reptiles and fish are another area of serious concern when they escape or are turned loose into non-native ecosystems by owners who no longer want them. If they survive — and that's a big if — they can spread disease and decimate local animal populations. For example, Burmese pythons set loose in Florida's Everglades National Park have bred for generations and nearly wiped out several species of native animals.

The bottom line: Keep your pets inside unless supervised. Indoor animals live years longer than their outdoor counterparts and do less damage to the environment around them. It's the greenest choice and the most ethically responsible.

4. Step 4: Remove Plastics and Chemicals

Many pet products made from plastics end up being trashed in the landfill each year. These nonrenewable materials can also be a danger to the health of you and your pet. Plastic pet products, including toys, beds, feeding bottles, bowls, and clothes, can contain polyvinyl chloride (PVC), a chemical classified as a human carcinogen and a danger to animal health by the US Environmental Protection Agency.[4]

Plastic feeding bowls and toys may also contain bisphenol-A (BPA), or include hazardous chemicals such as phthalates, a plastic softener that the Canadian Cancer Agency says has caused tumors in mice and lab animals.[5]

Avoid plastic whenever possible and opt for eco-friendly and renewable materials. Search for products that are BPA and phthalate-free.

Formaldehyde can be present in new fabrics and products such as pet beds, travel carriers, cushions, blankets, and clothing. It's best to wash new pet blankets, beds, and cushions before using — or leave them outside for a few days to air out and off-gas.

---

4 "Vinyl Choloride," US Environmental Protection Agency, accessed January 2016. epa.gov/airtoxics/hlthef/vinylchl.html
5 "Phthalates," Canadian Cancer Society, accessed January 2016. cancer.ca/en/prevention-and-screening/be-aware/harmful-substances-and-environmental-risks/phthalates/?region=on

4.1 Use your nose to sniff out toxins

Just like Toucan Sam used to follow his nose to find Froot Loops breakfast cereal, pet owners can sniff out toxins in pet products.

Lindsay Coulter, the "Queen of Green" at the David Suzuki Foundation, recommends doing a sniff test before buying plastic and fabric pet items, such as beds and clothing: Those that have a "new car" or "stinky" odor may contain phthalates and Volatile Organic Compounds (VOC).

"Many new products, from furniture to rugs and new clothing, have conventional finishes, seals, and paints that contain concentrations of VOCs," Coulter says. "Smell before you buy and avoid the headache. I mean that literally."

The Queen of Green recommends asking store owners and managers to carry no VOC or low-VOC products. And if the product stinks, leave it in the store.

4.2 Plastic bags

Millions of plastic bags used to collect pet waste, litter, and cage bedding end up in landfills every year and can take anywhere between 10 and 1,000 years to break down.

Whether you're using a bag to clean birdcage droppings or collect dog poop, do the environment a favor by choosing an eco-friendly alternative:

- Reuse a grocery store plastic bag that would have otherwise been thrown away.
- Brown bag it: Use a paper bag made with postconsumer material.
- Buy bags that are biodegradable or compostable.

4.3 Search for sustainable products

There are many great eco-friendly alternatives to plastic. Reduce your pet's "eco-paw print" by purchasing toys and products created using naturally sourced materials or recycled and post-consumer materials. Some, such as wicker, can be composted with your yard trimmings.

What these products are packaged in is equally important: Look for paper packaging consisting of 100 percent recycled paper.

Natural materials include:

- Organic cotton
- Bamboo
- Canvas
- Hemp, produced without herbicides and pesticides

- Natural rubber
- Untreated wood or bark
- Wicker

Sustainable and recycled materials include:

- Toys made with 100 percent recycled plastic
- Toys that can be recycled
- Upcycled products created with recycled goods
- Paper litters created with post-consumer newspaper
- Eco-fiberfill beds and stuffed animals
- Recycled water bottles (see below)

There are many North American manufacturers making great strides to divert plastic from our landfills by creating stylish and eco-friendly pet products using recycled plastic water bottles.

Montana's West Paw Design has diverted nearly 10 million plastic bottles from landfills by recycling them into what it calls IntelliLoft Fiber Fill and batting, which is used to stuff beds and plush toys for dogs and cats. The bottles are cleaned and striped of labels before being chopped into flakes, liquefied, and re-engineered into a nontoxic, sustainable, and recycled material.

The company has also pioneered what's hailed as an "infinitely recyclable" low-waste dog toy made from Zogoflex, a fully recycled (but super tough) material that's BPA and phthalate-free, and nontoxic. When you mail in your worn-out toys, the company recycles them into a new item, and that new item can in turn be recycled again into another toy — so the more products that are returned, the greener they become.

5. Step 5: Think before You Buy

Purchasing sustainable and eco-friendly pet products is a step in the right direction, but avoiding unnecessary purchases is the greenest choice of all.

The American Pet Products Association found that owners will spend $47 on dog toys and $28 on cat toys in a given year. But it's important to step back and evaluate what that item's purpose is and whether it is truly needed. Many dogs prefer chewing a stick outside to elaborate chew toys while cats will ignore a new treat and sit in the cardboard box it arrived in.

Before you make your next purchase, use Checklist 1 to decide whether you really need it so it doesn't needlessly end up in the landfill.

An easy way to reduce unnecessary toy purchases for dogs and cats, and to prevent boredom at the same time, is to limit the amount of toys they have access to at one time. Take half of their toys and put them in a storage box, and occasionally substitute them. The item brought back into rotation will be a "new" toy to your pet without ever having to make a purchase.

Pets are happiest spending time with their humans, so dedicating quality time to their exercise, enrichment, and companionship will do much more than any treat or toy you purchase.

Checklist I
Should I Buy It?

- ☐ Will it last a long time?
- ☐ Is it durable?
- ☐ What is it made out of?
- ☐ Does it contain toxic chemicals?
- ☐ How will I dispose of it?
- ☐ Can it be recycled?
- ☐ Do I really need it?
- ☐ Will this enrich my pet's life?

6. Step 6: Recycle

Just as we reduce our ecological footprint by donating and recycling items we no longer use around the home, we can do the same for our pets.

All across North America, there are city-run pounds and animal shelters that run on volunteers and limited resources to house homeless pets, and can't afford to spend money on luxuries for the animals housed there.

By donating your gently used pet and household items to your local shelter, rescue organization, or wildlife rehabilitation center you can make a double difference: Giving those items a new life while also making a big difference in your local community.

The following are some great items to donate to shelters and rescues:

- Harnesses, leashes, and collars
- Crates, carriers, and cages
- Aquariums
- Grooming supplies
- Newspapers to line cages
- Brooms, dust pans, and mop buckets
- Smart toys or Kongs
- Stuffed animals
- Towels and blankets

7. Step 7: Shop Locally

The "farm to fork" food movement has hit the pet world, and the environment is better for it. By choosing to buy pet food and other products locally instead of ones imported from another country, you are reducing environmental harm while also stimulating the local economy and helping the people in it.

The closer to home that products are manufactured, the smaller environmental footprint they create because they require less fuel-guzzling and carbon-polluting transportation to reach you. The production and shipping processes also require a great deal of packaging, much of it non-recyclable, if the products are being transported to far-flung markets.

Locally produced pet food and treats will be fresher and, in most cases, better quality: Vendors that sell directly to pet guardians require less additives and preservatives to retain the quality of their product.

Although it's not totally feasible to purchase all pet food and toys in your hometown, there are simple ways you can get involved in the locavore movement (locally produced food):

- Visit your local farmers' market for dog and cat treats and vegetable trimmings for your reptile, pig, rabbit, and other small pets.
- Ask your butcher for locally sourced meat and scraps, if your pet is on a raw diet.
- Buy hay for rabbits and pigs at a local farm feed store instead of at a pet supply store.
- Make a connection with a local farmer for bales of hay.
- Ask store staff where the product originated.

Even if you shop at big-box and department stores, you can still source local products. When you're looking at items, pay attention to where something is manufactured and the country it originated. There are many great North American companies that are producing nontoxic merchandise, and foods with wholesome ingredients.

Vote with your dollar: Ask the store manager if he or she can stock more local pet products. If more consumers request products that haven't traveled a long distance, the stores will respond by stocking them. Make your consumer dollars count!

8. Step 8: Buy Big

Making the choice to buy pet food in bulk is an eco-friendly triple whammy. It reduces vehicle trips to the store, reduces the amount of disposable packaging, and saves you money as the largest size is almost always the least expensive per unit. The bigger the order the bigger the discount.

If you have multiple pets or friends with the same type of pet consider contacting the food supplier or manufacturer directly to purchase food by the pallet. The bonus: They'll usually deliver it for free.

The only caution about buying big is ensuring that you can use all of the product before it goes bad. Check the expiration date.

9. Step 9: Make Your Containers Count

While many commercial pet food bags are made of paper, they are often lined with plastic or a nonrenewable coating to retain product freshness, so they can't be recycled. When you're buying bags of food check to see if they can be recycled or returned to the manufacturer for another use.

Phase out plastic when it comes to pet food. Start with what you use to carry and store pet treats. Instead of a plastic bag, use reusable bags and Tupperware instead.

Most big-box and conventional pet stores still use plastic bags at the checkout so bring your own reusable shopping bags when you visit the store to reduce your plastic consumption. If you have to use regular plastic bags, try to reuse them several times before discarding them.

10. Step 10: Get on the DIY Train

Homemade pet toys are an eco-friendly and inexpensive way to provide entertainment without spending money on nonrenewable products that will end up in the landfill. Remember, the best way to entertain and enrich your pets is giving them your time and attention, which doesn't cost a penny or require purchasing any product.

The following are a few ideas for every type of pet. (**Note:** Each individual animal chapter also contains great ideas to create enrichment items by repurposing everyday items in your home.)

Dogs:

- Tuck a recycled water bottle inside an old sock and knot the end. Dogs love the crinkling sound of the bottle being crunched and will happily munch away at it for days. When it's worn out, toss the old bottle in your recycling and sub in another.
- Cut an old shirt or sweater into strips and braid it to make a tug-of-war rope toy.

Cats:

- Shaker bottle: Put a marble inside an empty medicine bottle (ensure cap is tightly closed).
- DIY scratching pad: Loop lengths of rope around a thin board of untreated wood and hang on the doorknob or closet.
- Grow organic catnip in your yard.

Rabbits:

- Stuff Timothy hay inside used paper-towel rolls to make a chewing tube.
- A cardboard box with a doorway cut into it makes a great burrowing and hiding home.

Mini Pigs:

- DIY rooting box: Take a wooden box and fill it with larger river rocks. Sprinkle the inside with Cheerios, pig chow, or air-popped popcorn.
- Empty water or soda pop bottles make great mini-pig toys — they'll roll around with them for ages.

Birds:

- Create treat bundles by wrapping a few bird-appropriate snacks inside a Kleenex. Hang from top of cage with single strand of raffia or rope. Birds will root and peck to get to the treats by shredding the paper.
- Wood-block foraging tool: Take a small piece of untreated wood and drill holes in it to hide treats. Hang it from top of the cage.

Lizards:

- Build a climbing gym inside their terrarium using tree branches connected with a thick string or rope. Use thick recycled cardboard to build platforms to make it more interesting. Can easily be reassembled in new formations.

Fish:

- Pottery bowls, pots, and ceramic mugs make great fish ledges and caves in home aquariums. Just make sure there is no soap or soil residue.
- Use Lego pieces to create an amazing house or castle where your fish can hide.

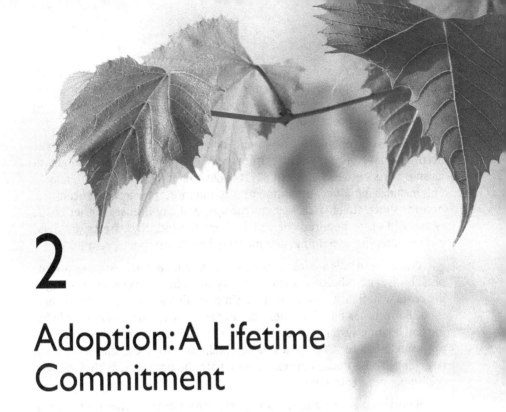

2

Adoption: A Lifetime Commitment

Falling in love with an animal is easy but taking care of it for life is much more difficult. Pets are our companions and family members. They boost our psychological, emotional, and physical well-being. However, being a guardian comes with a lot of responsibility and that aspect is often forgotten during the initial excitement of adoption.

Beyond the daily feedings and playtime, there are many hours of socialization and training required. Your new companion may need several hours of exercise daily to satisfy its physical and mental needs — not to mention saving your home from being destroyed by a bored and anxious animal.

Consider how many years that pet will be around. While dogs have a relatively short life compared to their human guardians, canines still live an average of 12.8 years, says Pets.ca.[1] Cats and snakes can live up to 20 years. And that's just a fraction of how long some birds live. Large parrots

---

1 "Tip 46 — Life Expectancy in Dogs — How Long Will My Dog Live?" Pets.ca, accessed January 2016. pets. ca/dogs/tips/tip-46-life-expectancy-in-dogs-how-long-will-my-dog-live

can reach 80 years of age, which is a concern because they may actually outlive their adopters. The Avian Welfare Coalition says all exotic birds, not just the bigger species, will be passed around to an average of seven different homes over their lifetime.[2]

Before you commit to a new pet it's a good idea to consider the costs. According to veterinary statistics from the ASPCA, the first year of pet guardianship costs between $235 to $1,314, depending on the type of animal.[3] This includes initial vet appointments, vaccinations, spay/neuter procedures, booster shots, training classes, microchips, and city licenses. Other costs, which add up to hundreds of dollars, include food, toys, treats, carriers, crates, boarding, grooming, and monthly health insurance premiums.

While these bills are less expensive for smaller animals, such as pocket pets, birds, and rabbits, it's worth noting that almost every pet has ongoing costs, whether it's for annual checkups or flea and tick prevention and food. For reptiles and fish, there are expensive and energy-sucking lighting and heating systems. The ASPCA says annual care costs range from $35 for a single fish to $300 for a small animal, $670 for a cat, and $875 for a large dog. Those dollar figures increase with the pet's age, as they require additional vet treatments.

Before you adopt a pet, it's important to consider whether the time is truly right to become a guardian. Ask yourself the following questions in Checklist 2.

I. Adopt Don't Shop

Money can't buy you love, unless you're using it to purchase a rescue pet. The most environmentally responsible pet guardianship decision you can make is adopting from a shelter or rescue instead of buying from a breeder or pet store.

By adopting you are not only saving that animal from certain death, you are also freeing up a space for another to be taken in. Only 29 percent of US pets are adopted from shelters and rescues, according to the ASPCA, while 2.7 million companion animals are euthanized each year.[4] By choosing adoption you are giving one of these great animals a second chance at having a love-filled life. Think of adoption as the "ultimate recycling."

I.I The horror of animal mills

There is a hidden dark side to the cute animal you see in the window of a pet store. Be it a pocket pet, rabbit, bird, snake, kitten, or puppy, animals

2 "Captive Exotic Birds: A Brief Introduction," The Avian Welfare Coalition, accessed January 2016. avianwelfare.org/shelters/pdf/NBD_shelters_introduction.pdf
3 "Cutting Pet Care Costs," American Society for the Prevention of Cruelty to Animals (ASPCA), accessed January 2016. aspca.org/adopt/pet-care-costs
4 "Pet Statistics," American Society for the Prevention of Cruelty to Animals (ASPCA), accessed January 2016. aspca.org/animal-homelessness/shelter-intake-and-surrender/pet-statistics

Checklist 2
Should I Adopt a Pet?

- ❏ How long will the animal live?
- ❏ How much free time do I have?
- ❏ Do I have someone who can help if I'm away or get sick?
- ❏ Can I afford the vet bills when the animal needs care?
- ❏ How large will this pet become?
- ❏ Will this type of pet be safe around small children and/or grandchildren?
- ❏ Is this pet a good fit for my life?
- ❏ Will my living circumstance change?
- ❏ Does this pet match my energy level and lifestyle?
- ❏ Would it be better for me to foster a pet before adopting permanently?

raised in commercial for-profit mills (e.g., puppy mills) contribute to the problem of pet overpopulation. These animals are raised in deplorable conditions without proper care for their welfare and health, not to mention the environment. Destined for pet stores in the US and Canada, mills and so-called "backyard breeders" produce litters of animals as quickly as possible in cramped, confined, filthy facilities, and they're shipped great distances in equally troubling conditions to reach the consumer marketplace.

Because their sole motivation is profit, mill operators and commercial breeders who sell to retail outlets and advertise on online marketplaces such as Craigslist and Kijiji do not care about the health and well-being of the animals, says Kathy Powelson, Founder and Executive Director of Paws for Hope Animal Foundation. As a result, many animals suffer long-term health problems and behavior issues.

Large-scale "factory-style" animal operations are also major polluters. A 2014 report by the US Humane Society found that because large amounts of feces, urine, and even animal carcasses are left on the ground for long periods of time, these facilities are a major producer of methane, a harmful greenhouse gas.[5] It's common for animals to become contaminated with pathogens because of the lack of basic hygiene and those toxins are transferred into soil — and drinking water — through their feces.

There are some pet retail chains that do adopt out animals in a humane, sustainable, and responsible way. PetSmart has pioneered adoptions from rescue groups in its more than 1,100 US and Canadian retail stores — with companion dogs and cats being provided by local animal welfare agencies and rescues. The company says about 7,000 homeless pets find new homes each week with the help of its 2,400 local adoption partners and donated retail space.

---

5 "Environmental Impacts of Puppy Mills," The Humane Society of the United States, accessed January 2016. animalstudiesrepository.org/hsus_pmc_rrafs/3

2. Breed-Specific Rescues

Maybe you loved the Siamese cats from *Lady and the Tramp*, or grew up with a Labrador Retriever and can't imagine your life without one. Perhaps you researched a specific breed of bird or reptile and decided it's the right fit for you and your family. No matter your reason for seeking a purebred, you don't need to go to the pet store or a breeder to get one.

To find your perfect purebred, start at your local animal control or city-run shelter. The myth that all animals in shelters are mutts or elderly — or elderly mutts — is completely untrue. Whether you're talking about dogs, cats, rabbits, or birds, the Humane Society says a full 25 percent of the shelter population are purebred.[6]

Use the website Petfinder.com to search for specific breeds based on where you live. This website is used by North American animal shelters and rescues alike to list all manner of animals big and small that need a forever home.

Another great source are breed-specific rescues focused on rehoming unwanted, abandoned, and homeless pets of a specific breed. These rescues are a responsible and green choice because by saving these animals you aren't contributing to pet overpopulation, and you are saving a life. These groups deal specifically with the breed you're interested in so they'll be able to provide great information about what to expect when it comes to their personality, temperament, training, and potential health issues.

All across Canada, the US, and the UK these groups, mostly volunteer run, specifically help match potential pet parents with their perfect purebred. The best resource to find a breed-specific rescue is the Internet, by searching the specific breed name plus "rescue."

The American Kennel Club provides a tool on its website to connect with 450 AKC Rescue Network groups across the US, representing 160 unique breeds (akc.org/dog-breeds/rescue-network). The Canadian Kennel Club does not have rescue clubs listed on its website; however, it is planning on adding them sometime in the near future (ckc.ca).

3. How to Find a Responsible Breeder

If you do choose to buy through a breeder, make sure it's an ethical one practicing sustainability who has animal welfare and the environment at heart. Ask questions, get vet records, phone references, and meet them in person. A red flag that an animal comes from an animal mill is a "breeder" that is unable to show you that young pet's parents or other littermates.

---

6 "Pets by the Numbers," The Humane Society of the United States, accessed January 2016. humanesociety.org/issues/pet_overpopulation/facts/pet_ownership_statistics.html

No reputable breeder would sell its animals to a pet store or puppy broker, says Kathy Powelson. In fact, the Canadian Kennel Club Code of Practice for breeders also prohibits its members from selling their dogs at pet stores.[7]

A good breeder will ask many questions of potential pet parents to make sure their animal is homed with a family that can provide affection and responsible care.

"Reputable breeders genuinely care for the animals they breed, and want to ensure that they are going to the best home possible so would insist on doing the screening themselves," says Powelson. "They often require a no breeding contract and will take the animal back at any time of that animal's life if their new owner is no longer able to care for them."

In its guide to finding a reputable and responsible dog breeder, the organization No Puppy Mills Canada recommends seeking someone who provides the following:[8]

- Belongs to a national or local breed club.
- Offers guidance, education, and support about the breed.
- Tests breeding stock for any congenital diseases and conditions, such as hip dysplasia.
- Produces vet paperwork.
- Immunizes puppies and has a spay/neuter contract.
- Shows the litter and "dam" — female parent — in a sanitary environment.
- Takes responsible care of its animals, including providing nutritious food, proper vet care, grooming, and socialization.

If a breeder doesn't live up to your standards, move on.

4. Short-Term Love: Fostering

Fostering is a short-term commitment that provides an animal love, comfort, and socialization in a temporary home while waiting for a permanent adoption. The pet gets much-needed human interaction and attention away from the stress of the shelter, while freeing up space for the facility to take in another animal. The welfare group fostering the animal will often pay for the food, supplies, and medical expenses while it is in your care.

Fostering is a great way to determine if you really want the full commitment of that type of pet, and whether that animal and breed is a good

---

7   Code of Practice for CKC Member Breeders, Canadian Kennel Club (CKC), accessed January 2016. ckc.ca/en/Breeding-Dogs/Code-of-Practice-for-CKC-Member-Breeders
8   "Reputable/Responsible Breeder," No Puppy Mills Canada, accessed January 2016. nopuppymillscanada.ca/NPMC%20Reputable%20Responsible%20Breeder.pdf

match for your home, family, and lifestyle. You get to shower that pet with love and attention, but it's a limited time before it is rehomed.

Sherri Franklin, the Founder and Executive Director of Muttville, a San Francisco-based group focused on improving the lives of senior dogs through rescue, foster, and adoption, says some of its volunteers have fostered more than 100 dogs before they ultimately gave a single dog its furr-ever home.

"Fostering a dog in need is a responsible choice that fulfills many foster family's hearts," Franklin says. "The more foster homes we have the more we can save."

Franklin admits some of its fosters are "foster failures" who permanently adopt the animal after seeing how well it does in the home, but that's a responsible choice too because it saves their life.

Animal shelters and rescue groups are always looking for volunteers to foster temporarily. To foster an animal, inquire with your local shelter or rescue group. You can also follow local animal groups in your area on Facebook, Instagram, and Twitter to receive updates about pets in need of foster homes.

5. Microchipping and City Licenses

Despite efforts to keep them safe, millions of North American pets get separated from their families each year and end up at animal shelters. Only a fraction are happily reunited. The ASPCA says only 26 percent of stray dogs are returned to their owner. For cats it's even worse: Just 5 percent find their family.[9]

There are inexpensive and easy ways to increase those odds. The first is a city license. Registering means officials will be able to easily and quickly find you should your pet wind up in "animal jail." This is extra crucial in overcrowded and underresourced facilities, where animals without identification could be euthanized or rehomed within several days if the owner can't be contacted. Many cities legally require a license, and it must be renewed annually.

A secondary method of pet identification is microchipping, a simple and relatively painless procedure that typically costs between $25 and $50.

The electronic chip, which is the size of a single grain of rice, contains your pet's identification and is implanted under its skin with a needle, usually between the shoulder blades. The chip, which can also record important medical history and information, such as allergies or medications, contains Radio Frequency Identification (RFID) and can be read by a scanner

---

9 "Pet Statistics," American Society for the Prevention of Cruelty to Animals (ASPCA),
   accessed January 2016. aspca.org/animal-homelessness/shelter-intake-and-surrender/pet-statistics

at a vet's office or shelter. **Note:** It's important to keep your personal information such as your phone number and home address in the chip updated with your veterinarian; otherwise, the device is useless.

The microchip is vastly superior to ID tags on a collar because the owner can still be tracked when the animal slips out of a home or yard when it's not wearing visible identification. And it lasts for the lifetime of the animal. The BCSPCA says pets implanted with a microchip are 20 times more likely to be reunited with their guardian.[10]

10 "Microchipping and Your Pet," BC SPCA, accessed January 2016. spca.bc.ca/assets/documents/welfare/microchipping-and-your-pet-1.pdf

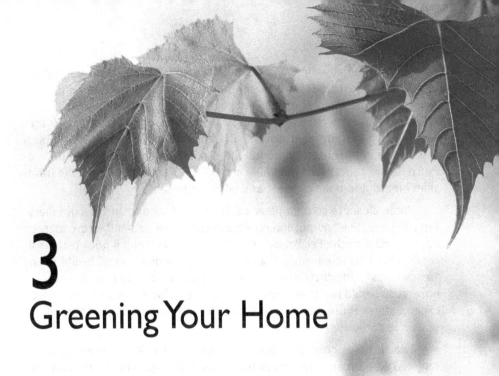

3
Greening Your Home

From chemical household cleaners to lawn fertilizers, some common household items are potentially dangerous to our companion animals — and the environment. This chapter discusses potential areas of harm and provides green alternatives.

1. Household Cleaners That Are Toxic to Pets

Just as some common household cleaning products contain ingredients that have potentially negative effects on human health, they can also be harmful to animals. With our pets spending much of their time on our floors and furniture, it's extra important to avoid using chemicals that could potentially hurt them. Curiosity coupled with cluelessness means animals have a much higher likelihood of ingesting products that can make them sick, and because of their small size and faster metabolism they can be poisoned by a very small amount of toxins.

"They groom themselves using their mouths, so residues from cleaning products and other environmental toxins end up in their skin, coat, eyes, nose, and throat," says Alicia Sokolowski, President of AspenClean, an eco-friendly house-cleaning service.

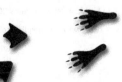

A 2008 study by the Environmental Working Group found alarmingly high levels of toxic chemicals from household cleaners in household pets. Blood and urine samples of cats and dogs were contaminated with 35 and 46 chemicals, respectively, including carcinogens, chemicals toxic to the reproductive system, neurotoxins, and endocrine disruptors. The group was particularly concerned about the carcinogens because dogs have a much higher cancer rate than humans: Up to 25 percent of dogs die from skin, breast, and bone cancers, as well as Leukemia.[1]

Home cleaners containing acids, bleach, ammonia, and glycol ethers can have negative and potentially deadly effects on pets if they are ingested, according to the Pet Poison Helpline, a 24-hour animal poison control center that's handled more than a million poisoning cases. While most "ready-to-use" products you buy at retail stores are diluted and would only cause a mild reaction, such as skin or eye irritation or stomach upset, experts stress those items need to be used properly to ensure the safety of pets in the home.

Bleach, toilet bowl cleaners, detergents, and grill and oven cleaners can lead to corrosive injuries in both cats and dogs. These products are especially hazardous to cats if they walk through an area wet with the detergent and lick their paws and groom themselves after. Similarly, the vapors left behind when using these products can be a skin and eye irritant, even in very small doses.

The following sections discuss common household cleaners that the Pet Poison Helpline says can cause harm.

1.1 Corrosive products: Drain and toilet bowl cleaners

Acidic products in the home such as drain, oven, and toilet bowl cleaners and anti rust compounds can result in severe poisoning, ruptured intestines, and most commonly, burns and tissue injury.[2] These products are typically bitter to taste and cause immediate pain when they contact your pet's mouth or skin. Pets can be harmed by drain and toilet cleaners when they drink water from the toilet. That's also why pet owners, in particular dog owners, should never use slow-release cleaning capsules in their toilet tanks. Close the toilet lid to ensure pets don't drink from it.

"These products are designed to be thick and eat away at the grunge but they can cause burns on the mouth and throat and esophagus," says Dr. Charlotte Flint, senior consulting vet for the Pet Poison Helpline. Pets usually drink from the toilet or lick the product out of the sink when their owner leaves the room when they're in the middle of cleaning.

---

1 "Polluted Pets," Environmental Working Group (EWG), accessed January 2016. ewg.org/research/polluted-pets
2 "Acids," Pet Poison Helpline, accessed January 2016. petpoisonhelpline.com/poison/acids

1.2 Detergents and laundry pods

Detergents aren't just what you use to wash dishes and clothes, they're also contained in many other household products, such as soaps, general cleaning sprays, and fabric softeners.

Cats are more sensitive to the phenols contained in these products. These can cause corrosive injuries. Residue from laundry detergent on clothes and sheets can irritate a pet's skin. Use all-natural formulations where possible.

Laundry pods are ultra-concentrated detergent packages designed to deliver a powerful punch of chemicals and can lead to drooling, vomiting, breathing issues, and coughing if dogs chew or swallow them. That's a problem because they're extra attractive to canines, says Dr. Flint: "Dogs seem to think they're fun to chew on and they tend to pop when they're chewed."

1.3 Floor cleaners

Pine oil, an essential oil that is used in floor cleaners and furniture polish, is poisonous and causes corrosive injuries to both cats and dogs. The biggest danger is if any cleaner is left on the floors and pets walk through it and lick their paws. It turns that dermal exposure into an ingestion injury.

1.4 Bleach, dishwasher detergents, oven cleaners

Unlike acids, which burn on contact, alkaline products such as bleach cleaners, automatic dishwasher detergents, and oven cleaners have little smell, taste, or odor, so pets are more likely to ingest a larger amount. Exposure can cause a range of caustic injuries from mild tissue irritation to eye and skin injuries. Thankfully, the majority of these exposures are minimal. If a dog chews on a bottle containing these products it can end in gastrointestinal and respiratory distress. If a dog chews or eats an alkaline dry cell battery, it can cause deep penetrating skin and mouth ulcers.[3]

1.5 Deodorizer sprays

The respiratory systems of birds are extremely susceptible to pump and aerosol deodorizer sprays, including perfumes and hairsprays, so take caution if you're using these around their cages. The same goes for the fumes from self-cleaning ovens and nonstick cooking surfaces: Both can be toxic to birds, according to the ASPCA. Sprays used around aquariums can pollute the water and cause distress. Consult Chapter 10: Birds and Chapter 12: Fish for a full list of household products that can cause harm.

A database of household chemicals hazardous to animals is available on the Pet Poison Helpline's website (petpoisonhelpline.com/poisons).

---

3 "Alkalis," Pet Poison Helpline, accessed January 2016. petpoisonhelpline.com/poison/alkalis

The following are ways to minimize harm to pets while using chemical cleaners:

- Sponge up any excess cleaner that pools on surfaces so pets don't lick it or walk through it.
- Follow directions as advised by the manufacturer.
- Keep pets off surfaces, especially floors, until they are dry.
- Keep bathroom doors shut if using drain and toilet bowl cleaners.
- Use products in a well-ventilated area.
- Put products away promptly when you are done in an area pets can't reach.

2. Eco-Friendly Retail Cleaners

There are many great household cleaners on the market that will leave your house sparkling without the use of noxious and potentially hazardous chemicals. Seek cleaning products labeled "nontoxic" and "organic." Be wary of products labeled "natural" because the term is not regulated, meaning anyone can use it to sell their product. Use unscented soaps and products to reduce the risk of skin irritation for your pet.

The following are several nontoxic brands of household cleaners that work well for general chores, pet odors, and messes:

- **AspenClean:** The Environmental Working Group (EWG) gave this line of nontoxic products straight A's in its Guide to Healthy Cleaning. These Ecocert-certified vegan products, voted product of the year in 2015, work hard and smell fantastic thanks to their essential oils. The ingredients are free from petrochemical surfactants and petroleum by-products and the bottles are made from at least 50 percent postconsumer resin. Available at Whole Foods and online at AspenClean (aspenclean.com/natural-cleaners).

- **Method:** Pet-friendly, naturally derived, biodegradable cleaners with packaging made from 100 percent recyclable material. Products include dish soap, floor cleaners, laundry detergent, and all-purpose cleaner. Sold in the US and Canada at most grocery stores and pharmacies.

- **Nature's Miracle:** This product is nontoxic, phosphate-free, and offers enzyme-based products for deep carpet cleaning and stain removal for messes from birds, cats, ferrets, dogs, and more. It also offers cage cleaners and general skunk odor removers. Sold in US pet stores or online (natures-miracle.com).

3. Go Green When You Clean: Make Your Own Cleaners

Better yet, you can create your own nontoxic household cleaners and de-odorizers that don't risk the health of your pet and your family. You can easily make great hardworking formulations with ingredients you already have in your kitchen cupboards, such as baking soda, lemon, olive oil, and nontoxic dish detergent. There's a hidden bonus: In addition to making your home sparkly you will also save money. Homemade cleaning formulas cost a fraction of their retail counterparts, and last many months.

Green cleaning begins with the tools you use to clean your home. Instead of cleaning up pet messes with disposable paper towels, use rags. If you're concerned about cross-contamination, cut up an old towel or dishcloth and designate it as the "pet mess" cloth and store it in a separate space. For general cleaning, use microfiber cloths. They'll last for years and are machine washable.

Pet-friendly cleaning supply kit:

- Nontoxic dish soap.
- White vinegar.
- Baking soda: This inexpensive staple is a natural odor absorber and carpet deodorizer.
- Table and Epsom salts.
- Hydrogen Peroxide (3 percent).
- Organic coconut oil.
- Rosemary and lavender oil: For fragrance, antibacterial, and antiviral qualities. You'll find this at your local health store.
- Lemon: Bottle of lemon extract is okay, or use freshly squeezed fruit.
- Spray bottles, microfiber cloths, microfiber rag mop, and ringer bucket.
- Pumie Scouring Stick: This 100 percent pumice product can be used to clean stubborn hard-water and rust stains in sinks, toilets, and tubs. You can use it wet on ceramic tile and it won't scratch.

The download kit that came with this book contains eco-friendly household cleaner recipes provided by Crystal Brisson, of Absolutely Clean Personalized Housekeeping Services, an eco- and pet-friendly cleaning company. The formulations include a hardworking general household cleaner, carpet deodorizer, grout cleaner, shower spray, and more!

4. Green Your Plants

Plants and flowers add green to your home and freshen the air, but did you know many common houseplants and flowers contain toxic substances that can be harmful to your pet's health if ingested? The US Humane Society has identified more than 700 hazardous plants. While the majority only cause minor issues such as nausea and stomach upset, some can cause paralysis or even death.[4] Before you bring home a new plant, be sure it's one that won't harm your furry friend.

4.1 Pretty but deadly: Lilies

Toxic reactions to lilies are one of the most common calls at the Pet Poison Helpline, especially for cats, who can develop tremors or seizures and experience kidney failure from nibbling even a tiny piece of the pretty flower. Even if cats just walk through lily pollen and groom themselves afterwards, the odds are they'll get sick. The most dangerous varieties are those considered "true lilies," which include Daylily, Tiger, Asiatic, Japanese Show, and Easter lilies. Unsurprisingly, cat poisonings spike around the holidays (i.e., Easter and Mother's Day) when bouquets containing these sickening blooms are brought into the home.

4.2 Decorative danger: Sago palm

Sold as a decorative mini palm tree in retail outlets such as Ikea, Target, and big-box home improvement stores, this now common Bonsai houseplant is toxic to both cats and dogs, though felines don't eat as much as their canine counterparts. If a dog gets into it, the animal will start having diarrhea and vomiting and it can progress into liver failure in just one or two days because of its cycasin toxin, says Dr. Flint. The seeds and roots have the highest concentration.

4.3 The dangerous green: Marijuana

With the rising prevalence and decriminalization of both medical and recreational marijuana, it's worth noting how toxic the tetrahydrocannabinol (THC) in it can be to pets. Trupanion, a leading US pet insurance firm, saw a huge spike in claims in 2015 for dogs and cats that raided someone's weed stash. While dogs can show toxicity symptoms within a few minutes of inhaling smoke or eating weed, they're usually minor, and eating a joint won't kill the animal. The bigger danger is if pets get into marijuana butter or "edibles," which have a much higher concentration of THC, and can cause low-blood pressure and seizures. Trupanion's message? Stash the stash to keep your pet safe.

---

4   "Plants That May Poison Your Pets," The Humane Society of the United States,
    accessed January 2016. humanesociety.org/animals/resources/tips/plants_poisonous_to_pets.html?
    credit=web_id97497736

4.4 Most common dangerous plants and flowers

The following are some of the most common plants and flowers that have negative effects to our pets' health — and how it affects them:

- **Aloe:** Causes vomiting and tremors.
- **Amaryllis:** Toxic to cats and dogs. Causes vomiting, depression, and tremors.
- **Azalea:** Eating just a few leaves can lead to vomiting and diarrhea, and in severe cases, coma or death.
- **Chrysanthemum:** Containing lycorine, eating this flower causes abdominal pain, vomiting, hypersalivation, and loss of coordination.
- **Daffodils:** The flower, bulbs, and plants can cause vomiting and abdominal pain.
- **English Ivy:** Causes vomiting, diarrhea, and can lead to coma and death.
- **Lilies:** Toxic only to cats.
- **Lily of the Valley:** Cardiac glycosides in the plant can cause a drop in heart rate, diarrhea, and seizures.
- **Oleander** Leaves of this popular outdoor shrub are highly toxic and can cause cardiac problems and death.
- **Rhubarb:** Causes limb weakness, diarrhea, and difficulty breathing.
- **Tulips/tulip bulbs:** The toxicity is concentrated in the stems and are often ingested when dogs dig in the garden. Causes stomach tissue irritation and convulsions.
- **Yew:** Causes tremors, trouble breathing, and sudden death from acute heart failure.

For more information about dangerous plants and flowers, the Humane Society has a downloadable and printable list of all plants that are poisonous to pets (humanesociety.org/assets/pdfs/pets/poisonous_plants.pdf).

4.5 Pet-safe plants

There are many beautiful houseplants to brighten your space and improve your home's air quality that won't cause harm to your pets. Here are some of the most common houseplants that are nontoxic to dogs and cats:

- Areca or Golden Palm
- Bamboo and bamboo palm
- Blue Echeveria
- Bottle Palm
- Fern Holly or Japanese Holly

- Painted Lady (also known as Copper Rose)
- Haworthia
- Hens and Chickens
- Pearl Plant
- Reed Palm
- Spider Plant, Spider Ivy

There are hundreds of other healthy plant options for pets on the ASPCA's online database (www.aspca.org/pet-care/animal-poison-control/toxic-and-non-toxic-plants/b?&field_non_toxicity_value[01]=01&page=3).

5. Your Lawn and Garden

While most pet owners are concerned about the dangers of fertilizers and herbicides sprayed onto lawns, for the most part these only cause mild stomach upset, and only happen if the animal walks through the wet product. To keep your pet safe, make sure any of these products dry on your lawn before letting your pets on it.

The bigger concerns for garden products are insecticides, snail and slug killers, and vermin bait. Also note that just because you use organic products in your garden that doesn't mean they're pet-friendly. Blood and bone meals, compost piles, and naturally green lawn solutions can also be hazardous to your pet's health.

In the download kit you will find a pet-safe recipe for weed killer provide by Absolutely Clean Personalized Housekeeping Services.

5.1 Insecticides

Commonly mixed into herbicides and fertilizers used by flower and rose gardeners, insecticides that contain Organophosphates (OP) and carbamates are toxic to pets and can cause symptoms ranging from stomach upset to bloody vomit, pancreatitis, and comas. The Pet Poison Helpline says it records hundreds of calls annually about these products.

5.2 Snail and slug killers

It's very common for snails and slugs to invade gardens in some regions. Grub or snail killers containing metaldehyde are particularly poisonous. If dogs gobble up the granules, they can develop tremors and seizures. The ASPCA refers to this type of poisoning as "shake and bake" because it causes the animal's temperatures to shoot up rapidly — as high as 42.2 degrees Celsius (108 Fahrenheit).[5] Dr. Tina Wismer, from the American Society for the Prevention of Cruelty to Animals (ASPCA), says dogs will eat the whole box because they love the taste.

---

5 "Metaldehyde," Pet Poison Helpline, accessed January 2016. petpoisonhelpline.com/poison/metaldehyde

5.3 Gopher and mole bait

Bait is often put into gardens to prevent rodents from nibbling veggies. Baits containing phosphides can end up harming household pets. When ingested by your dog or cat, these poisons release toxic phosphine gas in the stomach, causing bloating, vomiting, seizures, and tremors. If that gas is expelled from your animal's stomach, it can affect people too.

"If they vomit, it becomes toxic to people. So people can inhale it if they're taking the dog to the vet and the dog farts in the car," says Dr. Charlotte Flint of the Pet Poison Helpline.

Keep the animals in a well-ventilated area and don't feed them if you suspect they've ingested the toxic bait.

5.4 Blood and bone meals

Bone, blood, and fish meals, commonly used as organic fertilizer to boost the nitrogen content in garden soils, taste delicious to pets because they contain ground up dried and flash-frozen animal bones. In fact, it's so appetizing that hungry dogs will gobble up several pounds of it, leading to a "cement-like" blockage in their gastrointestinal tract that may have to be surgically extracted.[6] A bigger issue is when these meals are mixed with insecticides, which can lead to toxic poisonings in cats and dogs.

5.5 Compost piles

A steaming garden compost heap can resemble an all-you-can-eat buffet for your pet. Although it's made of organic materials, these compost piles can produce hazardous mycotoxins if food or plant matter has grown mold. Eating those moldy items can cause vomiting, tremors, and seizures in pets, so make sure to keep your compost pile inaccessible to your four-legged loved ones.

5.6 Naturally green lawn solutions

Forget bugs and weeds, the biggest killer of any green lawn is your dog relieving itself on it. A dog's urine has a high nitrogen content so it causes burns, dead spots, and yellow patches when it comes into contact with the grass. One way to stop the scalding is to water the area immediately after your dog pees to dilute the concentrations of nitrogen, but that requires you following your dog around with a hose or bucket, which doesn't work if your dog is by itself in the yard.

There is a natural, eco-friendly solution that you can add to your pet's water dish that will stop urine burns. Dog Rocks is a natural rock mined from an Australian quarry that drops the nitrogen level in water so it won't be ingested when your dog drinks. Dog Rocks won't repair the grass that's

---

6 "Bone Meal & Blood Meal," Pet Poison Helpline, accessed January 2016. petpoisonhelpline.com/poison/bone-meal

already damaged, but it says you won't see any new dead spots and there will be a "vast improvement" in your lawn in five weeks. The natural rocks last for around two months, and cost $18.50 (dogrocks.org).

6. Pet-Proof Your Home

With all household chemicals and products that are hazardous to pet health, the most important thing is keeping them out of sight and out of reach from your animals. This is especially true for cats, who can jump onto upper closet shelves without a problem. Just as new parents prepare to baby-proof their home, animal owners must ensure their house is safe for their fur babies. Here are some considerations:

- Keep bottles containing chemical products and medications tightly closed.
- Follow directions carefully for cleaning products and make sure the area is well-ventilated when you use them.
- Mop up any excess moisture from products to reduce fumes.
- Keep your cleaners out of reach of pets. The same goes for body lotions, personal body supplies, and medicines.
- Keep a list posted in your home of the plants and foods that are toxic to pets.
- Keep the number of your vet and a pet poison hotline on hand in case of emergencies (see section 7.).

6.1 Garage

Commonly used to store automotive and garden items, the garage can be one of the most dangerous places for your pet. The following sections discuss some of the worst offenders, and some pet-friendly alternatives.

6.1a Sweet killer: Antifreeze

Dogs have a serious sweet tooth, and it's that attraction to sugary-tasting substances that leads to thousands of antifreeze poisonings in garages each year. Unlike some acidic products that burn on contact, antifreeze tastes good, so pets end up slurping up large amounts. Call it sweet but deadly: The ethylene glycol in it is toxic and it only takes a few tablespoons to "seriously jeopardize an animal's life," says the Humane Society of the US. It says a seven-pound cat can be killed just by drinking a single teaspoon.[7]

There is a pet-safer alternative. Vehicle owners can switch to a brand that contains propylene glycol instead of ethylene glycol. It's still toxic, but much less so. The product can be slightly more expensive than its deadlier counterpart, but you don't need a lot for the whole season, so the

---

7 "Antifreeze Is a Sweet but Deadly Poison for Pets," The Humane Society for the United States, accessed January 2016. humanesociety.org/animals/resources/tips/antifreeze.html?referrer=https://www.google.ca

extra expense isn't a big hit to your pocketbook. Keeping your pets safe from antifreeze is easy: Always make sure to wipe up spilled product, and keep leftover fluid on a high shelf where pets can't reach it.

Windshield wiper and brake fluids containing the toxic alcohol methanol are also hazardous.

6.1b Mouse and rat poisons

Pet poisoning from so-called rodenticides is one of the most common and tragic calls the Pet Poison Helpline receives each year. Generally, there are two popular types on the market, both with their own inherent risks if your dog or cat gets into them. The first are anticoagulant rodenticides (ACRs), which cause internal bleeding in cats and dogs when ingested. These poisonings can be treated with a Vitamin K antidote, but thankfully instances of this type of poisoning are decreasing because of tighter restrictions on the products by North American regulatory agencies. The US Environmental Protection Agency halted the sale of eight common ACR products in 2015 after ruling the pesticides posed "unacceptable risks" to children and pets that came into contact with the bait.[8]

The much more serious poisoning comes from mouse and rat poisons containing bromethalin, which is toxic and has no antidote. These common products can cause brain swelling and neurological symptoms.[9]

For pet owners who have pest problems, there are nontoxic rodenticides on the market. Look for products in your hardware store that consist of "natural cellulose" from powdered corncobs. These corn or maize derived natural products work by essentially dehydrating the mouse or rat by interfering with their water absorption. They're nontoxic and don't pose a risk of poisoning "non-target" animals.

6.2 Bathroom

One of the most hazardous rooms to your pet's health is the bathroom, where animals can potentially access and ingest toxic cosmetics, beauty creams, and medications meant for humans. Ibuprofen is the second leading cause of pet poisoning in the home behind chocolate, according to the ASPCA Animal Poison Control Center. The candy coating present on many pills is irresistible to your dog's sweet tooth.

"Dogs love to play with the bottles but they also love the taste of it. We find dogs will eat more pills than cats will but it's dangerous to both," says Dr. Tina Wismer, the center's Medical Director.

That's not the only human medications pets are getting into: The poison center receives plenty of calls about painkillers (including aspirin and

---

8 "Canceling Some d-CON Mouse and Rate Control Products," United States Environmental Protection Agency, accessed January 2016. epa.gov/rodenticides/canceling-some-d-con-mouse-and-rat-control-products
9 "Mouse and Rat Poison," Pet Poison Helpline, accessed January 2016. petpoisonhelpline.com/poison/mouse-and-rat-poison

acetaminophen), cold medicines, anti-cancer drugs, antidepressants, vitamins, and diet pills — all of which can all be toxic to animals.[10]

Items that are commonly on countertops, such as mouthwash and toothpaste, can also cause a hazard because the fluoride in it is poisonous to both cats and dogs. A bigger concern is toothpastes and mouthwashes containing the natural sugar sweetener xylitol, which can cause life-threatening low-blood sugar in dogs, even in very small doses. Just like those candy-coated pain pills, dogs love the taste of xylitol because it's sweet. Dental floss can also be ingested and can get tangled in your pet's stomach.

To keep pets safe, keep medicine containers and tubes of ointments and creams away from pets who could chew through them, and be vigilant about finding and disposing any dropped pills.

7. How to Treat a Poisoned Pet

Pet poisoning can happen in a heartbeat. If you suspect your pet has ingested a hazardous household chemical contact your veterinarian or a poison control expert immediately. Be prepared to advise the expert about the following:

- What product the pet was exposed to and approximately what amount.
- How long ago it happened.
- Age, weight, and size of your pet.
- Symptoms the pet is displaying.

Signs of pet poisoning include vomiting, drooling, lack of appetite, difficulty breathing, diarrhea, listlessness, abdominal pain, muscle tremors, fever, and lack of coordination. The first few hours after poisoning are critical to your pet's survival and recovery, so getting in touch with a professional as soon as you know is key.

The following are hotlines that can provide immediate help, 24 hours a day:

- Pet Poison Helpline: 1-855-764-7661 (petpoisonhelpline.com). A $49 fee, payable by credit card, applies. This covers an initial consultation and follow-up calls. The staff provides advice for poisoning cases of all species, including dogs, cats, birds, small mammals, large animals, and exotic species.
- ASPCA Animal Poison Control Center: 1-888-426-4435 (aspcapro. org/poison). A $65 consultation fee may be applied.

---

10 "Common Household Dangers for Pets," The Humane Society of the United States, accessed January 2016. humanesociety.org/animals/resources/tips/common_household_dangers_pets.html

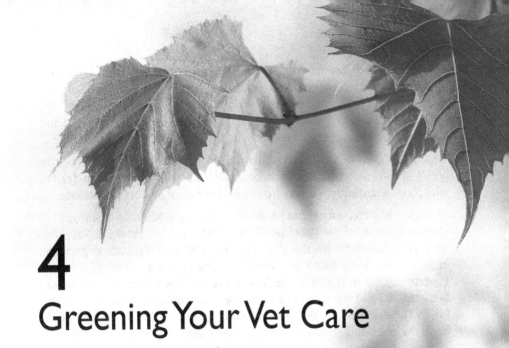

4
Greening Your Vet Care

Veterinary treatment for pets is big business: The American Pet Products Association estimates animal owners spent $15.7 billion on vet care in 2015, with annual costs hovering around $200 for the average dog or cat owner.[1] This chapter examines how you can lower the environmental impact of your pet's vet visits, and how to use preventative care to keep your animal healthier, so it requires less of medical interventions.

1. Don't Contribute to Pet Overpopulation

The number one thing you can do to reduce your pet's environmental footprint is to have it spayed or neutered. To say that North America has a pet overpopulation problem is an understatement. The American Society for the Prevention of Cruelty to Animals (ASPCA) says there are 70 million stray cats in the US alone. More than 7.6 million companion animals end up in American animal shelters each year including a staggering 3.9 million dogs and 3.4 million cats.[2]

---

1 "US Pet Industry Spending Figures & Future Outlook," American Pet Products Association (APPA), accessed January 2016. americanpetproducts.org/press_industrytrends.asp
2 "Pet Statistics," American Society for the Prevention of Cruelty to Animals (ASPCA), accessed January 2016. aspca.org/about-us/faq/pet-statistics

Their futures are far from bright: 41 percent of cats and 31 percent of dogs that enter shelters are euthanized simply because there are not enough homes for them, and shelters don't have enough resources, says the ASPCA. More than 2.7 million shelter animals will be killed in 2016 alone, roughly one animal every 13 seconds, according to the US Humane Society.[3]

At the core of this overpopulation problem are dogs and cats that aren't sterilized, but also small pets such as rabbits, rats, and ferrets, which can sire multiple litters from a young age in a short time frame.

A single intact animal can produce a shocking amount of offspring in its lifetime because of the multiplier birth effect. Seattle's Feral Cat Spay/Neuter Project teamed with the University of Washington's math department in 2009, and using data from North Carolina feral cat colonies, academic experts calculated that a single female cat and her offspring will produce between 100 and 400 kittens in seven years, provided the adult cat lives that long.[4] The experiment illustrates an alarming number, and just how out of hand the pet population can become if animals aren't spayed or neutered.

1.1 Health benefits of spaying and neutering

Altering an animal will help it live a longer life, with less likelihood of needing toxic and chemical-laden medicines, veterinary interventions, and chemotherapy associated with cancer treatments. Because the ovaries and testes are removed during the procedure, sterilizing greatly decreases, if not completely eradicates, the odds your animal will become sick with any illnesses linked to its reproductive tract. In fact, sterilizing a dog will increase its life by an average of one to three years, and prolong the life of a feline from three to five years, according to SpayUSA, a US nonprofit service for affordable spay/neuter services.[5]

For altered female cats and dogs, the risk of breast, ovarian, and uterine cancer, as well as mammary gland tumors, is a fraction of what it would be, says SpayUSA. For male dogs and cats, it says the low-risk, low-cost surgery eliminates the risk of testicular cancer, and also greatly lowers the likelihood of prostate disease. There are also positive side effects for behavior: Neutered male dogs display less aggression and dominance, bite animals and people less frequently, and have a reduced risk of being injured in fights or vehicle accidents because they have less desire to roam.

The American Veterinary Medical Association (AVMA) says the health benefits of sterilization are increased if it's completed before the first heat cycle, adding that it can also protect female dogs and cats from uterine infections later in life.[6]

---

3 "Pet Overpopulation," The Humane Society of the United States, accessed January 2016. humanesociety.org/issues/pet_overpopulation/?credit=web_id80597225
4 "How Many Kittens in Seven Years?" *Feral Cat Times*, Feral Cat Spay/Neuter Project, accessed January 2016. feralcatproject.org/documents/newsletters/feb_06newsletter.pdf
5 "Benefits of Spay/Neuter," SpayUSA, accessed January 2016. spayusa.org/benefits.php
6 "Spaying and Neutering," American Veterinary Medical Association (AVMA), accessed January 2016. avma.org/public/PetCare/Pages/spay-neuter.aspx

Because cats and dogs as young as five months old can get pregnant, SpayUSA recommends that animals undergo the procedure before six months of age. It says the average age for spay/neuter is four months. Consult your vet to determine what the most appropriate age is to alter your pet.

2. How to Find a Great Veterinarian

Choosing a vet is a personal decision, but one of the most important to make sure your pet lives the healthiest life possible. You want to find someone who you trust with your animal and believe will provide the highest quality of care. The following are some easy tips to find the best vet for your pet:

- **Ask around:** Ask friends, family members, coworkers, and other pet owners for recommendations.

- **Call breeders and rescue organizations:** Groups that specialize in working with a specific animal have a lot of interactions with vets, and often have great input on who has the best price, service, and conduct. Your city-run animal shelter is also a good source of information.

- **Go online:** Professional organizations including the American Animal Hospital Association and Canadian Veterinary Medical Association have directories of accredited vets and hospitals on their websites. Certification in these organizations is not mandatory in all states and provinces but it does denote high standards for patient care, record keeping, and training. Look at the Google and Yelp reviews of the clinic to see how actual pet guardians rate their professionalism and animal care.

    - American Animal Hospital Association: aaha.org/pet_owner/about_aaha/hospital_search/default.aspx

    - Canadian Veterinary Medical Association: canadianveterinarians. net/membership/directory-vets-hospitals

- **Seek a specialist:** The physiology of companion animals is very different so it's not realistic to think that all veterinarians have the same knowledge base when it comes to small animals, reptiles, and birds. That's why it's important to seek a specialist, or an exotics vet, to ensure your pet is treated by someone who is experienced in treating that type of animal. It also reduces the chances your pet will be given unnecessary or inappropriate medical treatments.

- **Visit the practice:** Ask for a tour of the clinic. See how the vets and technicians interact with other staff and the animals in their care. Ask questions and don't be afraid to ask for referrals from other pet owners. Find out if the clinic provides emergency care. If you don't get a good feeling about the practice, move on.

Many veterinary clinics have green protocols in place to minimize their impact on the environment, from how their office is run to how hazardous materials are disposed of. Ask your vet if there is a policy in place to reduce the impact of veterinary medicine on the environment. This could include waste disposal, recycling, high-efficiency lighting, cleaning agents, and biosecurity protocols.

3. Alternative Medicine: Holistic Vet Care

As the popularity of holistic therapy rises for people suffering from chronic illnesses and health conditions, more pet owners are turning to alternative therapies for their veterinary care. Under its umbrella of treatments, including acupuncture and chiropractic, holistic vets say they can ease and resolve animal health issues such as digestive upset, allergies, diabetes, and geriatric problems, including arthritis and joint pain. Its natural interventions for acute and chronic diseases substitute eco-friendly homeopathic and natural pain remedies for conventional medicines and therapies that use toxic chemicals and often have harsh side effects.

Jill Elliot, Doctor of Veterinary Medicine (DVM), a leading holistic vet in New York City, said treating animal cancer patients with homeopathy gives the vast majority a better prognosis — without the invasive chemical treatments.

"Without any chemo or radiation it will give them the same life span as the chemo promises, and they'll be happy and healthy and have more energy during that time," Dr. Elliot says.

Homeopathic remedies are naturally derived from plants, animal products, and minerals. Its focus on preventative care makes homeopathy and holistic care an eco-friendly alternative to pumping your pet full of drugs when it experiences issues, and can serve as a natural complement to traditional veterinary medicine.

4. Vaccinations

Vaccinating your pets boosts their immune response and creates antibodies to protect against contagious and deadly infectious diseases. It helps their bodies fight off infections that can cause serious illness. Generally, the first set of vaccines are given within six months of an animal's life, with the first set of boosters given a year later.

There are currently no vaccinations recommended for rabbits, hamsters, rats, mice, Guinea pigs, gerbils, or snakes. For cats and dogs, the American

Veterinary Medical Association (AVMA), American Humane Association, and Canadian Veterinary Medical Association (CVMA) agree there are standard core vaccines needed for both animals.

The following are essential vaccines for dogs:

- **Rabies:** The rabies virus can strike all mammals, including humans, and is nearly always fatal. Vaccination against rabies is required by law in most US states and Canadian provinces.

- **Distemper:** Often called the distemper shot, the DHPP vaccine prevents against hepatitis, parvovirus, and parainfluenza. Distemper, spread through eye and nose discharges of infected animals, causes nervous system and respiratory issues in dogs and is fatal in about half of cases. Parvovirus, spread through infected feces, causes vomiting and severe diarrhea and can cause death in as little as 48 hours. Parainfluenza is one of the causes of kennel cough, which is a hacking cough and includes flu-like symptoms.

The following are essential vaccines for cats:

- **Rabies:** The rabies vaccination is required by law in most US states and Canadian provinces. The CVMA recommends indoor cats get inoculated because they may sneak outside, or rabid wildlife, such as skunks or raccoons, can get into a fenced yard.

- **Feline viral rhinotracheitis, calicivirus, and panleukopenia (PVRCP):** Commonly called "feline distemper," this vaccination protects against three diseases. Panleukopenia is a potentially lethal viral disease that causes diarrhea, dehydration, and sudden death, while rhinotracheitis and calicivirus infects the airways of felines, and can cause cold-like symptoms and mouth ulcers.

Your vet may recommend additional vaccinations for your pet depending on the following:

- Age and lifestyle.
- Geographic area.
- How much time it spends outside.
- Number of animals in the home.
- Travel and kenneling.
- If you visit off-leash parks, pet daycares, and boarding kennels.

5. Hidden Dangers of Flea and Tick Medications

The most readily available treatments to eradicate fleas and ticks in both cats and dogs are also the most controversial and potentially hazardous to your pet's health. In 2009, the US Environmental Protection Agency (EPA) issued a harsh warning over the use of approximately 70 so-called "spot on" flea and tick control products because of a spike in adverse reactions.[7] The chemical liquid insecticide treatments are squirted directly onto the animal's skin, usually between the shoulder blades, to prevent larvae from hatching and also act as a neurotoxin to the blood-sucking parasites.

The EPA's report was shocking: 43,000 adverse reactions were reported in a single year for cats and dogs using the popular products, including skin irritation, vomiting, tremors, gastrointestinal distress, nervous system issues, and 600 deaths. The products contained the active ingredients cyphenothrin, pyriproxyfen, phenothrin, S-methoprene, permethrin, and dinotefuran, among others. The EPA found that dogs younger than three years old and small dogs less than 20 pounds were more likely to have adverse effects. Miniature Poodles, Pomeranians, Chihuahuas, and Bichon Frises were overrepresented in the sicknesses. The government agency concluded that weight ranges listed on the products might be too broad, meaning the tiny canines got a too-high dose. Despite the tens of thousands of negative health effects reported, the products remain on the market, and are still sold at most pet stores. The EPA reported a high number of incidents with the misuse of permethrin dog treatments in cats, despite labels that warned against the treatments being used on felines.

Acknowledging that popular pet store flea and tick medications can cause animal illnesses, Health Canada issued an alert in 2015 advising consumers on the safest way to use the products:

- Always follow the directions on the packaging.
- Only use the amount specified on the instructions based on the size and weight of the animal.
- Never apply the insecticide on animals younger than the minimum age stated on the product.
- Never use on different animals (e.g., dog products on cats, and vice versa).
- Report any negative health effect to the manufacturer.

See the download kit for natural solutions for fleas and ticks.

6. Preventative Medicine: Annual Checkups

Just like you take your car in for a tune-up, your pet benefits from an annual checkup to detect health problems and act as a starting point for preventative care.

During the physical exam a veterinarian can detect any changes in the animal's overall health and look for signs of age-related illnesses such as dental disease, heart problems, and diabetes. An animal-care professional

---

7 "US and Canada to Increase Scrutiny of Flea and Tick Pet Products," United States Environmental Protection Agency (EPA), accessed January 2016. yosemite.epa.gov/opa/admpress.nsf/ eeffe922a687433c85257359003f5340/cb98fe802d1162a78525759a00686ef0!OpenDocument

can detect things that you may not, such as irregularities in blood pressure or a heart murmur. This is also the time to examine whether your pet's vaccinations are up to date and whether a booster is needed. Use this time with your vet to bring up any other issues or concerns, including behavioral, food counseling, and weight management, or any health problems your pet's breed may be genetically prone to.

7. How to Dispose of Unwanted Medications

Despite our valiant efforts to keep them safe and healthy, in your pet's lifetime you will likely find yourself with prescription and over-the-counter medications for animals in your home that will need to be discarded. The issue is that these chemical-laden medications can pose a risk to pet, human, and environmental health if they are disposed of improperly. Here's what to do with them:

- **Don't flush:** Never flush unused pharmaceuticals down a drain or toilet. The majority of water-treatment facilities and septic tanks aren't designed to filter out contamination from chemicals, so flushing medications means they will end up in your community's water system. This has potential negative consequences not only for the people who drink the water, but the waterways themselves. Pharmaceutical pollution in rivers, streams, lakes, and oceans can hurt the water's eco-system, which has negative effects on its fish and wildlife.

- **Follow vet instructions:** If you receive prescription medication from your vet, closely follow the instructions on how to administer it. Animal-care experts optimize medicine quantities to ensure pet health and to reduce expense to the pet owner, so there should be very few unneeded doses at the end of treatment. If your pet is prescribed medicine, speak to your vet about what you should do with any leftover doses.

- **Return them:** Never throw medications, syringes, or needles into the trash. Instead, return them to your veterinarian for proper disposal. In the US, vets need authorization from the state to collect and dispose of unwanted or expired medications, according to the American Veterinary Medical Association. It recommends disposing of pharmaceuticals through authorized take-back events, mail-in programs, and collection bins.

8. Slim, Trim, and Happy: Avoiding Pet Obesity

The North American obesity epidemic isn't limited to people. In its eighth-annual National Pet Obesity Prevalence Survey, the Association for Pet

Obesity Prevention (APOP) found that a whopping 58 percent of cats and 53 percent of dogs in the US were overweight. Of these, 17.6 percent of dogs and 28.1 percent of cats were classified as obese, which means they were more than 30 percent over their ideal body weight. More troubling is that the survey revealed that the vast majority of owners had no idea.

It found that 90 percent of owners of overweight cats and 95 percent of owners of overweight dogs believed their pet was a normal weight.[8] Researchers coined this the "fat pet gap," a phenomenon that's concerning because obesity is the number one health risk faced by pets. Just like obesity in people, extra weight on pets leads to massive health problems that can bring a lifelong dependence on unnecessary medications.

Problems associated with obesity in dogs can start when the animal is just five pounds more than its ideal weight, according to the association, and weight issues can shave years off your pet's life, not to mention add up to thousands of dollars in unnecessary vet bills. The Canadian Veterinary Medical Association (CVMA) says obesity can lead to a laundry list of health issues including high blood pressure, diabetes, arthritis, reduced liver function, and heart problems. The CVMA says overweight pets are 50 percent more likely to develop cancer, and fat animals are at much greater risk during surgery and recovery because of reduced lung, kidney, and liver function and extra pressure on their heart and arteries.[9]

It's not just dogs and cats: Birds, reptiles, fish, pigs, and small animals are also prone to packing on the pounds.

The APOP created an online obesity translator that compares the weight of obese pets to portly people in a bid to demonstrate how serious extra weight is on a small animal (petobesityprevention.org/how-fat-is-that-doggie-in-your-window).

Take a look at the following examples:

Yorkshire Terrier

With an ideal weight of 8 pounds, if a Yorkie is 4 pounds overweight (a total of 12 pounds), it is 50 percent overweight. The human equivalent is a 5'4" woman weighing 218 pounds (73 pounds overweight) or a 5'9" man weighing 254 pounds (85 pounds overweight).

(petobesityprevention.org/wp-content/uploads/2010/07/Yorkshire-terrier.pdf)

---

8 "US Pet Population Gets Fatter; Owners Fail to Recognize Obesity," Association for Pet Obesity Prevention, accessed January 2016. petobesityprevention.org/u-s-pet-population-gets-fatter-owners-fail-to-recognize-obesity
9 "Obesity Poses Serious Health Hazards to Pets," Canadian Veterinary Medical Association (CVMA), accessed January 2016. canadianveterinarians.net/documents/obesity-poses-serious-health-hazards-to-pets

Domestic shorthair cat

With an ideal weight of 8 to 10 pounds, if a cat is 10 pounds overweight (a total of 18 to 20 pounds), the human equivalent is a 5'4" woman tipping the scales at 290 pounds (145 pounds overweight) or a 5'9" man weighing 338 pounds (169 pounds overweight). Each extra pound on a cat is equal to an extra 15 on an adult woman or 17 on a man, according to the APOP's calculations.

(petobesityprevention.org/wp-content/uploads/2010/07/Cat.pdf)

The APOP estimates that owners overfeed their pets by as much as 25 percent. The biggest problem is the "eyeball effect": Instead of portioning out meals in a measured fashion, many pet owners judge the portion size by how much it fills the bowl, or "eyeballing" it. The result? Way more food ends up in the serving dish than what's actually recommended and they get a "super-sized" meal. The same result happens when pets, especially cats, are allowed to use so-called "self feeders" that dispense kibble whenever it's desired.

Most of the time the real problem lies with how animals tug at our heartstrings: Despite our pets being a fraction of the size we are in terms of weight, we have the tendency to feel bad about the (relatively) small amount of food we give them for a meal because we are subconsciously judging that portion size against what it would take to fill our own stomachs. It's the same anthropomorphizing that happens when we give our pets an extra helping of food because they are begging, or we perceive they are giving us a sad look. Both scenarios go against the veterinary evidence that tells us the proper calorie intake pets need to live a healthy, long life without becoming obese and in need of medical treatment.

The simplest and most effective weapon in the war on pet obesity is a measuring cup. Always feed pets based on their weight and follow the manufacturer packaging directions. If you're unsure, consult a veterinarian about what an appropriate portion is for your pets' current weight, or, if they're overweight, how much they should be fed to reach their ideal weight.

Watch those treats! Pet treats are a huge and hidden source of daily calories for a pet, especially one that is overweight, elderly, or leads a sedentary lifestyle. A single treat can be the pet caloric equivalent of a human having a hamburger or a slice of pie. Treats should not make up more than 5 to 10 percent of your pet's daily caloric intake.

How to reduce treat calories:

- **Give sparingly:** A treat really should be used as a "treat" and not given in multiples.

- **Split them up:** A single Pup-Peroni pepperoni-style dog treat has 24 calories. If you cut it into four pieces, that's a much more reasonable 6 calories apiece.
- **Opt for healthier treats:** Look for low-calorie treats in your favorite pet store, or opt for healthier foods that you already have in the fridge, such as mini carrots or pieces of cooked chicken. In the summer, freeze chicken broth into ice cube trays for a refreshing treat.

(See more about healthy treats in the chapters about individual pets.)

9. Consider Pet Insurance

Aging pets require more medical treatments, even if they're healthy, which can translate to thousands of dollars in vet bills that can catch you off guard. Cancer treatments for animals can easily soar to $5,000 and higher. For a small monthly premium, pet insurance can help cover large medical bills down the road, should your companion animal become ill, get injured, or require costly surgery. Coverage plans vary dramatically and may not cover all conditions and bills so it's important to do your homework before signing on with a company.

Premiums vary based on species, breed, age, and how comprehensive the coverage is. Plans may include deductibles, co-payments, exclusions, and have payout limits. As an add-on service, some insurance companies offer "Pet Wellness Plans" that cover routine and predictable expenses such as teeth cleaning, vaccines, and flea medications.

An alternative to insurance is setting aside a predetermined amount of cash each month into a savings account to help defray vet bills down the line. With standard deductibles of $250 and reimbursement levels hovering around 80 percent, this may be a better option from a financial standpoint. However, this option does require a lot of discipline.

10. The Greenest Goodbye: Humane Euthanasia

The cruelest injustice of being a pet owner is that most companion animals live a much shorter life than their owners. Humane euthanasia is the most compassionate option when the animal's quality of life deteriorates because of age or illness and it is beyond treatment. Although it's heart wrenching to say goodbye, it's unfair to prolong your ill or elderly pet's life and subject it to more pain, suffering, and invasive medical interventions.

There is never a perfect time, so get the opinion of your veterinarian. Even though it's difficult, be with your pet when it is put to sleep. The presence of a vet in your pet's final hours can make it fearful so the most compassionate thing to do is to be there.

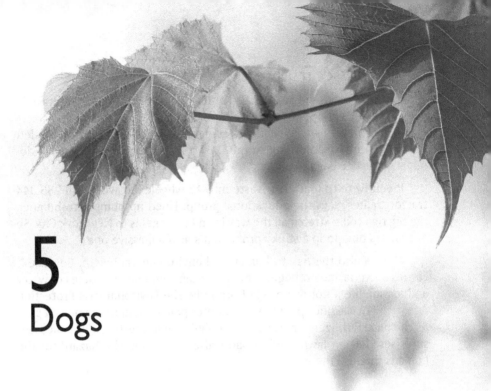

5
Dogs

With 86 million dogs in North America alone, it's no doubt that they are man's best friend. However, between their meaty diets, chemical grooming products, plastic toys, and poop, our canine buddies can also be the environment's worst enemy.

While canines used to be relegated to the backyard eating table scraps, our relationship with dogs has changed in recent decades. They are no longer just pets: Many believe they are family members, and with that new title comes an increase in spending. Americans shelled out an estimated $60.59 billion on pet products in 2015, everything from specialized diet food to memory foam beds and dog clothes.[1]

All that consumption doesn't necessarily give your pet a better life. In fact, canine obesity rates are at an all-time high because we are providing too much food and decadent treats and not enough exercise. This chapter discusses easy strategies that will not only reduce your dog's carbon paw print but also enhance and lengthen the life of your four-legged friend.

---

1 "Pet Industry Market Size & Ownership Statistics," American Pet Products Association (APPA), accessed January 2016. americanpetproducts.org/press_industrytrends.asp

1. The Stinky Truth: Dog Poop

One of the biggest and stinkiest dilemmas dog owners face is what to do with their pet's poop. In America alone, 22.9 trillion pounds of dog waste is generated every single year — a staggering percentage of which is left on the ground — according to the Doody-Free Water Project, which donates pet waste bags to parks.

If you were to load that waste into 18-wheelers it would fill 286,344 tractor-trailers, says the educational group. Lined up bumper-to-bumper, the big rigs could stretch all the way from Los Angeles to New York City. So not only is dog poop a stinky problem it's also a massive one.

There's also the risk to human and environmental health. Because it carries bacteria and pathogens, pet feces can contaminate bodies of water and marine life if not disposed of properly. The Environmental Protection Agency (EPA) classifies pet waste as a water pollutant, in the same category as chemical fertilizers, motor oils, and faulty septic systems.[2] "Unpleasant surprises" left on lawns and in parks also create a health hazard for the humans that use them.

The 411 on Dog Poop

- 340 grams: How much waste a typical dog produces per day, according to an EPA study on water pollution.

- 684 pounds: How much waste a single 100-pound dog will generate in one year, according to the Flush-Doggy.com poo calculator.

- 50,000 pounds: How much pet waste is generated every single day in Seattle, Washington.

- 97,000 tonnes: How much dog feces end up in regional parks in the Vancouver, British Columbia, area each year, according to Metro Vancouver.

- 62.7 million pounds: How much poop the Doody-Free Water Project says is created by US dogs every single day.

- 730 bags: Number of extra plastic bags in the landfill each year if your dog poops twice a day and you dispose of it in a bag.

- 1,000 years: How many years it takes for a conventional plastic bag to break down in a landfill.

---

2 "What Is Nonpoint Source?" United States Environmental Protection Agency (EPA), accessed January 2016. water.epa.gov/polwaste/nps/whatis.cfm

- 23 million bacteria: Number of fecal coliform bacteria in a single gram of pet waste, which is the size of a pea.

1.1 How to dispose of dog waste

The impact of your dogs' waste on the environment is related to their size: Obviously, a Great Dane will excrete exponentially more poop than a tiny terrier or Chihuahua. No matter your pets' stature, or how many you own, you are totally in control of their environmental harm:

- **Pick it up:** The easiest and most effective way to curb environmental contamination is to scoop the poop! Contrary to the belief that rain will just wash away the waste — and the hazards within it — that's simply not true. Dog poop that's not cleaned up is carried into storm drains and drainage ditches and is swept untreated into lakes, rivers, and streams, where pathogens can end up harming human drinking water supplies. The high nitrogen content in pet waste depletes oxygen in the water, which has devastating effects on the fish and other marine wildlife. In many cities it's not a question of pet owner responsibility — it's also against the law not to pick it up.

- **Collection services:** If you're not a fan of picking up dog poop, there are many dog-waste collection companies that will do it for you for a small monthly fee. It also diverts waste from the landfill: Most services will transport it directly to a local waste-treatment facility. To find one in your area search "dog waste collection" online. Hiring a service is a good option for pet owners with limited mobility or apartment and townhouse complexes that can share the cost.

- **Flush it:** Flushing the poop allows it to be properly treated at a local waste treatment facility or sewage plant, and eliminates the potential for it to contaminate soil and water. Many municipalities prefer this option. Use caution if you flush the baggies: Even those labeled "flushable" can cause clogs in your home plumbing and city sewers.

Generally speaking, biodegradable bags can be flushed but compostable ones can't because they need heat to break down. The David Suzuki Foundation warns pet owners to be wary of "degradable" bags because they contain formulated polythene, which leave small pieces of plastic in the water when they fragment.[3]

- **Compost it:** You can easily convert dog waste into organic fertilizer for your flower and ornamental gardens by composting it along with your green waste. Some cities even accept pet waste in

---

3 "Disposing of Dog Poop the Green Way," David Suzuki Foundation, accessed January 2016. davidsuzuki.org/what-you-can-do/queen-of-green/faqs/waste/disposing-of-dog-poop-the-green-way

compostable bags along with food and green waste in municipal compost environments, so check your local bylaws. Never use dog waste compost on food crops. (See the download kit for instructions on how to build your own dog-waste composter.)

- **Throw it out:** Depending on your local city bylaws, you can throw small amounts of pet waste into your household garbage. Because it can pose an environmental hazard in landfills, and release methane gas, this should be used as a last option after flushing and composting. The most eco-friendly way to discard poop is in a biodegradable or compostable bag — regular grocery bags take exponentially longer to break down, which halts the composting process altogether.

- **Green bag it:** Whether you are planning on flushing the poop, throwing it out, or composting it, opt for a green bag whenever possible for collection. Choose a compostable or biodegradable bag over regular plastic bags. Even a paper bag, preferably made from postconsumer materials, will break down much faster.

There are many great biodegradable and compostable pet waste bags available at pet stores and big-box retailers that are made from renewable and plant-based materials, such as vegetable starches. These bags break down when exposed to heat, oxygen, and mechanical stresses.

In order for a product to be officially certified as compostable and biodegradable under the strict ASTM D6400 standards in the US, the bags must be proven to break down in every type of landfill environment within a specific time frame and leave no harmful residues behind.

There's a catch: The lack of moisture in landfill piles slow down the organic decomposition process, making it nearly impossible for many bags to live up to those tough standards. So even though some nontoxic pet waste bags aren't government certified as biodegradable they will still break down exponentially faster than plastic bags and release no harmful chemicals into the atmosphere, making them a better choice.

What to look for in a green poop bag:

- **Plant-based:** Look for starches created from non-GMO crops, such as tapioca and corn.

- **Core:** Many bags that are sold in rolls contain a core. Look for cores made from recyclable cardboard instead of plastic.

- **Scented versus unscented:** Bags scented with synthetic fragrances can contain toxic chemicals that are released as the bag decomposes. Look for unscented bags, or companies that use natural fragrances, such as lavender.

- **Packaging:** Look for products sold with minimal packaging made from postconsumer materials.
- **Dispensers:** Poop bags often come in plastic dispensers. Look for ones that are made from number 5 plastic that can be added to your home recycling bin, or sent back to the company for recycling.

The following are some retail recommendations:

- **PoopBags:** This Chicago company produces poop bags made from plant matter such as corn, vegetable oil, and compostable polymers, including some that are 100 percent biodegradable and have the highest ASTM D6400 certification. The orange-scented PoopBags are made from 30 percent postconsumer material and its poop bag dispensers are made from almost 40 percent renewable resources. They are available online at PoopBags.com, at Petland in Canada, and several thousand independent pet retailers in the US.

- **Earth Rated Poop Bags:** Costing just pennies per poop, these tough, leak-proof green-colored bags are available in lavender-scented and unscented options and contain an additive from Environmental Technologies Inc. (EPI) that helps them break down faster than a traditional plastic bag. Also available are white-colored vegetable-starch bags that meet ASTM guidelines and can be composted. Earth Rated's dispensers are made from recyclable plastic. Sold in major pet stores in the US and Canada and online through Amazon. For more information go to EarthRated.com.

2. Dog Food Dilemma

With sales of dog food expected to reach $14-billion in the US alone in 2016, it's easy to see why the pet store aisles are packed with a dizzying array of products, promising everything from a softer coat to stronger teeth.[4] However, determining which food is the most nutritious for your four-legged friend — and what it's made of — is difficult.

While packaging uses images of premium cuts of meat, whole grains, and farm-fresh vegetables those are rarely what's inside the bag. Many commercial dog kibbles contain rendered by-products from factory farming, including meat trimmings, animal remnants, and even dead and diseased livestock — all deemed unfit for human consumption.

"These scraps are ground, heated, and mixed with cereals and soybeans colored to make them appealing to the human eye, sprayed with flavorings to make them palatable and then preserved," says Marcella Paraskevas-Ramirez, a holistic animal practitioner and educator in New Jersey.

---

4 "The United States Pet Food Market," Agriculture and Agri-Food Canada, accessed January 2016. agr.gc.ca/eng/industry-markets-and-trade/statistics-and-market-information/by-region/united-states/the-united-states-pet-food-market/?id=1423068874885

The super heating and cooking process of rendering is designed to kill harmful pathogens and bacteria, but recent widespread pet food recalls involving contaminated ingredients, including the 2007 melamine contamination that caused 14 pet deaths, prove that the process isn't foolproof.[5]

There are also environmental and health fears about the hormones and antibiotics used in US livestock and chemical pesticides and fertilizer for plants that legally ends up in the food we feed our dogs.

"All the concerns that apply for the human food chain also apply to pet food," says Sabine Contreras, canine nutrition consultant and owner of Better Dog Care, whose website, The Dog Food Project, helps consumers make informed pet food decisions.

The biggest driver of change in the pet food industry is our own dietary preferences. As health-conscious consumers seek food that is minimally processed with less chemicals and environmental impact, we demand those products for our pets as well. The 2014 Canadian Pet Market Outlook found that 21 percent of dog owners are likely to spend more to get healthier, higher-quality foods for their dogs — and agree natural and organic products are superior.[6]

While it's tempting to choose a food that mimics our own personal eating preferences (e.g., grain or gluten-free, or added probiotics and omega-3), some fad ingredients don't have significant health value to our four-legged friends.

No matter what kind of food you choose to give your dog (e.g., freeze-dried, kibble, wet food, homemade, or raw), there are ways to reduce the associated carbon footprint, and optimize their health in the process. Just as we understand that minimally processed, whole foods are better for us than junk food and prepackaged meals, the same is true for our pets. Ask questions about what's in your dog's food, including where it comes from and what it's made with. If you're not satisfied with the answer, buy elsewhere. You vote with your consumer dollars.

There are many easy ways to lower your dog's food footprint, including:

- Cut down on packaged food and treats.
- Use durable feeding bowls: Choose stainless steel over plastic and china.
- Control portions: Feeding in excess is wasteful and creates obese pets that require more vet care for weight-related issues.
- Feed meat-free treats, such as carrots and roasted sweet potatoes or biscuits.

5 "Charges Filed in Contaminated Pet Food Scheme," US Food and Drug Administration, accessed January 2016. www.fda.gov/ForConsumers/ConsumerUpdates/ucm048139.htm
6 "Consumer Corner: Canadian Pet Market Outlook, 2014," Alberta Agriculture and Forestry, accessed January 2016. www1.agric.gov.ab.ca/$department/deptdocs.nsf/all/sis14914

- Feed less beef: Cattle production is the most polluting and environmentally draining of all animal proteins.
- Use naturally shed antlers for treats (see section 5.1).

There is no single food that is the best for every dog. Consult with your veterinarian or a canine nutrition specialist to seek the best diet plan for your canine's age, weight, health, and activity level.

2.1 Decoding mysterious labels

In the US, dog food is regulated by the Association of American Feed Control Officials (AAFCO), a voluntary organization that establishes pet food safety regulations. In Canada, there is no equivalent agency. The labeling of pet food is regulated by Industry Canada, and the Pet Food Association of Canada (PFAC), a group of manufacturers, which says it complies with its voluntary guidelines.[7]

Understanding pet food labels isn't simple. Some items, such as weight, need to be backed up with standards, but others don't. For that reason, labels aren't a good indicator of whether the dog food is healthy.

"The label does not tell consumers what is being used," says Susan Thixton from the association for Truth about Pet Food. "Consumers are not told if they are buying a 'chicken skin and bones' pet food or a 'chicken meat from a USDA-inspected and approved for human consumption' pet food. It's all a big mystery."

The biggest weapon consumers have in the fight to find eco-friendly and healthy food is knowledge. Being able to decode labels will allow you to cut through the marketing buzzwords and determine what will actually enhance your dog's health — and curb its environmental impact. The following are the Association of American Feed Control Official's (AAFCO) legal labeling standards:[8]

- **Ingredients by weight:** Packaging must display all ingredients in decreasing order by weight, meaning the biggest contributors are the first items. Manufacturers aren't required to list what the percentage of each ingredient is, so if the first ingredient is meat but the second and third are grains, it could mean there is more grain than animal protein in the food. Similarly, if an ingredient is at the end of the list, it is likely not enough to make a significant difference in the nutrition.
- **Complete and balanced:** This label means the food meets a certain AAFCO standard for "nutritional adequacy" and can be fed daily. This doesn't mean optimum nutrition or speak to the quality of the food,

---

7 "Industry Regulations," Pet Food Association of Canada, accessed January 2016. pfac.com/industry-regulations
8 "What Is in Pet Food," Association of American Feed Control Official (AAFCO), accessed January 2016. aafco.org/Consumers/What-is-in-Pet-Food

just that it meets the minimum standard for nutrients for a dog's different life stages (i.e., growth, reproductive, and maintenance).

- **Natural:** The AAFCO definition is very broad; generally speaking, this means food that does not contain artificial and chemical additives, preservatives, and colors. There is no requirement for natural ingredients to be safer or more nutritious than those produced with chemicals.

- **Premium, super premium, holistic:** These terms are essentially meaningless. They have no legal definition and do not speak to the nutrition or quality of the product.

- **Organic:** Administered through the National Organics Program, the ingredients may not contain synthetic fertilizers, sewage sludge, irradiation, and genetic engineering. Certified organic pet foods must display a United States Department of Agriculture (USDA) organic label and contain at least 95 percent organic ingredients.

- **Human-grade:** For a pet food to be classified as human grade, manufacturers must prove to the USDA that everything is "edible" by human food standards, which is an expensive and arduous task. Very few pet food products are certified human-grade.

- **Meat:** Primarily animal flesh but can also include less appealing cuts of meat, such as the heart. Bones are not allowed to be added. The "meat" can come from cows, pigs, sheep, or goats, but it must be identified if it comes from another animal, such as buffalo, fish, or chicken.

- **Meat and animal by-products:** Meat deemed unfit for human consumption, either for aesthetic reasons or because it is parts of the animal people would not eat. That includes, but is not limited to, lungs, udders, brain, blood, spleen, bones, and intestines. The species of animal must be listed unless it is from cattle, pigs, sheep, or goats.

- **Meat and bone meal:** Highly processed and rendered by-product that can contain organ meat, trimmings, and bones. This can legally include so-called "4D" (i.e., animals: dead, diseased, dying, and disabled). There are certain things not allowed into meal by law, such as hides, hair, hooves, or horns, unless what may occur "in good processing practices," says AAFCO.

2.2 Rendering: The ultimate recycling?

Animal protein rendered into dog food is a controversial but hugely important topic. Renderers collect 56 billion pounds of animal material in North America each year, according to the National Renderers Association.[9] Nine

---

9 "Rendering Is Recycling," National Renderers Association, accessed January 2016. d10k7k7mywg42z. cloudfront.net/assets/53e623d1f002ff3e7c00027c/infographic_brochure_web.pdf

billion pounds are made into animal feed and pet food through the rendering process, which removes fat and water and cooks it into a "meal."

The majority of animal protein used in commercial pet foods is a natural by-product or secondary product of human food manufacturing that would otherwise end up in the landfill or incinerator, says the National Renderers Association, which is why the association says it's a sustainable pet food choice. It argues if all rendered products were thrown away, all available landfill space would be used in four years.

Feeding your dogs more of these "recycled products" is a great way to lower your pet's carbon footprint, says Jan Jarman, a commercial feed consultant and a representative of The Association of American Feed Control Officials (AAFCO) Pet Food Committee.

"There is a 'yuck factor' in rendered products. But the meat and bone meals are required to be safe, they would be prohibited from commerce if they were not," she says.

It's worth noting that not all animal protein used in pet food is rendered. A representative of AAFCO says ingredients such as meat meal, fish meal, poultry meal, and meat and bone meal are rendered, while ingredients such as meat, poultry, fish, meat by-products, poultry by-products, and fish by-products are not.

The National Renderers Association says rendered animal protein can legally include animals that are too sick to be sold as human food, livestock that die in transit on their way to the slaughterhouse, and expired grocery store meat. Pet food advocates say more insidious things routinely end up in the renderer as well such as roadkill, dead zoo animals, and euthanized cats and dogs from shelters.

The shock and yuck factors aside, from a purely environmental standpoint using waste from a system that produces excess biomass could be seen as a reasonable way to use the large volumes of usable (but unpalatable) animal protein.

2.3 Raw diets

The popularity of feeding dogs a diet of raw meats, bones, and vegetables is soaring. Proponents say dogs are evolutionarily built to eat raw meat, and tout a range of benefits including shinier coats with less shedding, healthier skin and teeth, better breath, smaller poops, and increased energy levels. They believe feeding uncooked meats, whether it's home-prepared, freeze dried, or commercially purchased, can curb chronic digestive issues, ear infections, allergies, arthritis, and obesity. The diets include mineral-rich organ meats, such as kidneys and livers, and muscle meat and bones, either whole or ground.

"Raw meat contains a lot of protein and is rich in many other nutrients such as enzymes, minerals, vitamins, and essential fatty acids that are needed by dogs," says Marcella Paraskevas-Ramirez, a holistic animal practitioner and educator in New Jersey.

From an environmental standpoint, feeding raw has two benefits, the first being that your dog will produce less biological waste. The reason for that, advocates say, is that because you're feeding smaller amounts of pure protein and veggies with no grains, filler, and by-products, more of the nutrients are absorbed directly into the body instead of passing through it.

Raw diets can also have a tinier environmental footprint because you can purchase the food from smaller companies that source all of their meat, vegetables, and bones locally, versus using an international brand whose product is shipped around the globe

"Quality lamb, for example, is almost always from New Zealand, while other exotic meats like Kangaroo and Alpaca, must be shipped in to match," says Brian Feldbloom, owner of Naturally Urban Pet Food Delivery. "Supporting locally made products is a great way to cut down on the energy used to produce and distribute."

The American Animal Hospital Association and Canadian Veterinary Medical Association both caution pet owners against feeding raw, saying any perceived benefits are outweighed by the potential health risks for pets and their owners when it comes to the pathogens in raw meats, and potential for contamination. However, believers say those risks are virtually eliminated by proper food handling.[10]

2.4 Becoming a natural dog chef

Just as we improve our health by decreasing our consumption of highly processed and packaged foods, some animal lovers believe the journey to optimum dog health starts with a diet of homemade food created with wholesome and natural ingredients.

With concerns over the quality and safety of the ingredients in commercial kibble, making your own meals means you control what your pup eats — and can ensure a diet free of chemicals and preservatives.

Generally speaking, homemade meals contain a protein source (i.e., meat, fish, dairy, plant-based), fat, carbohydrate, and vegetables or fruit. They can be cooked in large batches in the slow cooker, then frozen in reusable containers and thawed when needed.

Pet parents that want to feed homemade need to do their homework to ensure their dog's health isn't put at risk. Supplements, including calcium, need to be added to ensure the meals are nutritionally complete.

10 "Raw Protein Diet," American Animal Hospital Association (AAHA), accessed January 2016. aaha.org/professional/resources/raw_protein_diet.aspx#gsc.tab=0

The DIY diet is also inherently environmentally friendly:

- You can source your own local and organic meats and vegetables, which helps local farmers.
- No packaging: You are no longer buying bags and cans of food, which end up creating waste.
- No carbon emissions from shipping food products to your pet store.
- Containers: You can use your own glass containers to store the food.

There are hundreds of recipes for homemade dog food online, but anyone starting this regime for their dog should consult a canine nutritionist or vet before making major changes.

2.5 Veggie dogs?

Bramble the Border Collie, one of the Guinness World Records oldest dogs, lived to 27 years old on a vegan diet. The UK dog, who passed away in 2003, is often cited as a shining example of how canines can live — and thrive — without meat.

There's no doubt that removing meat from a dog's diet reduces its carbon footprint, and many pet owners are doing just that over concerns about the massive negative environmental impact of industrial farming and ethical and philosophical concerns about slaughtering and eating animals.

"Feeding companion animals plants instead of animals sends a market signal that consumers don't support the factory farming industry and the unnecessary killing of other animals," says author and animal activist Gene Baur, who founded Farm Sanctuary, where all resident animals eat plant-based diets.

The carbon footprint of meat-free diets consisting of plant proteins, whole grains, and produce is further reduced because most people opt to make the meals themselves, giving them the option to source non-GMO and local ingredients.

The concern is whether imposing our personal values on our dogs puts them at risk. Even companies such as VegePet, which sells a nutritional supplement to add to vegetarian and vegan pet meals, says dogs can end up malnourished and suffer serious health problems if their plant-based diet isn't nutritionally balanced and properly supplemented with vitamins, minerals, and calcium. A deficiency of the essential amino acids taurine and carnitine can lead to a type of heart disease known as dilated cardiomyopathy.

Some nutritionists believe it's okay to feed vegetarian, but stop short of veganism.

"If someone wants to feed their dog as a vegetarian, this diet should at least still include plenty of eggs and dairy protein, and ideally some wild-caught fish," says canine nutritional consultant Sabine Contreras.

VegePet says unlike obligate carnivores that require animal protein, such as cats, dogs are nutritional omnivores that can get all the nutrients they require through consuming plant-based proteins. While many denounce this theory, saying that dogs are actually natural carnivores, believers say a plant-based diet can improve the animal's energy level, skin, coat, and teeth while decreasing the risk of cancer, infections, and obesity.

Simply sharing your own food isn't enough though: Implementing a meat-free diet requires a great deal of research and planning, and should include meeting a canine nutritionist or vet before making any changes. The diet may not be suitable for young puppies or senior dogs.

3. Green and Clean: Eco-Friendly Grooming

Many grooming products contain harsh chemicals and synthetic colors, smells, and ingredients that are suspected carcinogens, irritants, and hormone disruptors. These can have negative health effects for both the dogs being cleaned and the humans that come into contact with them. Even if your pet is pampered in a salon, grooming chemicals are spread to pet owners when the dog returns home and snuggles with family and lays on furniture.

The problem isn't just surface level: An overlooked health issue is that animals absorb toxins through their skin and fur during grooming and ingest it as they lick to clean themselves afterwards, or lick and chew itchy spots.

"This means if you are putting a shampoo or coat conditioner on your pet that has harsh, toxic or carcinogenic chemicals in it, not only is your dog absorbing it all over their body, they are eating it as well," says Adam Coladipietro of Spa Dog Organic Dog Spa, an organic dog grooming studio in Vancouver, British Columbia.

Chemical-based grooming products are also a danger to the environment. Petroleum products washed down the drain can wreak havoc on marine ecosystems and pollute drinking water sources. By choosing products made with organic and natural ingredients your dog and Mother Earth will be nurtured. If you use a grooming service, look for one that only uses eco-friendly products. If it doesn't, ask if you can supply your own.

3.1 Decoding grooming product labels

There are few legal or regulatory requirements when it comes to the ingredient labels on pet grooming products. Try to source products from companies that voluntarily list ingredients — and ask a question if there's something you don't recognize.

Look for the following:

- Formulations that are biodegradable so they won't harm waterways and wildlife when they are washed down the drain.
- Products free of synthetic fragrances and parabens.
- Organic oils (e.g., coconut, olive, sunflower).
- Guar gum and citric acid used as thickeners.
- Scents that use organic essential oils (e.g., lavender, rosemary, mint, orange, and juniper).
- Vegan: Plant-based products always have a lower carbon footprint than animal products.
- Refillable or returnable containers.
- Packaging made from recycled and postconsumer materials that can be recycled.

The following "foul four" are the worst environmentally offending ingredients in dog grooming products, and should be avoided:

- **BHA (butylated hydroxyanisole):** Used as a preservative in dog shampoos, this synthetic antioxidant has been classified as a potential human carcinogen by the International Agency for Research on Cancer. It's been found to cause lung, liver, and kidney problems in lab animals and is banned in cosmetics in the European Union.
- **DEA (diethanolamine):** Used to make shampoos and soaps sudsy or creamy, cocamide DEA can cause skin and eye irritation and has been linked to liver cancer, according to the David Suzuki Foundation. The International Agency for Research on Cancer classifies DEA as a possible human carcinogen.
- **SLS (sodium laureth) or SLES (sodium lauryl ether sulfate):** These inexpensive foaming agents are the most common detergents in dog shampoos and can cause eye or skin irritation. The Environmental Working Group has linked SLS to organ toxicity, cancer, and neurotoxicity.
- **Synthetic colors and fragrances:** Meant to enhance the smell or color of a grooming product, many synthetics are created from petrochemicals. These can often contain aldehydes, benzene derivatives, and synthesizers that are known to cause allergic reactions, migraines, and asthma symptoms, according to a warning from the David Suzuki Foundation. Diethyl phthalate in synthetic fragrances is also harmful when it's washed down the drain, as it can be toxic to marine wildlife.

3.2 Retail grooming supplies

If you're buying your own grooming supplies, look for items made from sustainable materials with minimal packaging. For brushes, look for natural rubber and bamboo, and avoid plastic. Dog hair can be added to the compost bin.

The following are some recommended retail products:

- **Black Sheep Organics:** The ingredients used in its line of beautifully fragrant organic shampoos, bug sprays, ear wash, and toothpaste are certified organic or wild harvested. All products are biodegradable, vegan, cruelty-free, and a portion of the proceeds are donated to environmental organizations. Available in more than 50 stores in Canada, and online at BlackSheepOrganics.com.

- **Organic Oscar:** This line of shampoos, conditioners, pet wipes, and deodorizing sprays are organic and 100 percent biodegradable. The products do not contain any parabens, petroleum-based ingredients, dyes, or artificial fragrances. Available in US stores and online through OrganicOscar.com and Amazon.

The download kit contains a recipe for a nontoxic dog shampoo free of parabens and synthetic fragrances. Recipe provided by Lindsay Coulter, the "Queen of Green," at the David Suzuki Foundation.

4. Flea, Tick, and Insect Control: The Natural Way

There are many effective chemical-free methods you can use to protect your dog from outdoor enemies, including mosquitos, ticks, and fleas.

Flea control inside the home:

- Bathe pets often using natural and organic products, or even a few drops of a nontoxic dishwashing liquid. Fleas can't hold onto your dog's hair shafts when they're wet, and they'll fall off into the water.

- Use a flea comb often, in between baths. If you catch any, flush them down a drain in hot water.

- Vacuum furniture and carpets often, and disinfect the floors using eco-friendly soap in hot water. Always make sure to empty the vacuum canister — and take it outside — so that the fleas don't live on inside the vacuum and reproduce.

- Wash bedding often — theirs and yours. Always use hot water.

Outside the home:

- Give your pet a full body check after being in wooded areas or parks.

- Trim the lawn. Ticks can hang out in tall grasses and will latch onto passing animals.

- Reduce exposure to mosquitoes by eliminating standing water in your yard.
- Keep your pets indoors at dusk and early morning when the mosquitos can be the worst.

Natural repellants:

- Only use pesticide and chemical-free flea, tick, and mosquito repellents for pets.
- Buy a natural flea collar that uses a blend of essential oils instead of potentially toxic chemicals.
- Add a natural repellent to the outside of your dog's collar. In its guide to nontoxic flea removal methods, the Natural Resources Defense Council recommends essential oils made with lemongrass, cedarwood, peppermint, rosemary, or thyme, which you can purchase in a natural health store. A few drops of geranium, cedarwood, and lavender oils on your dog's collar will act as a natural bug-stopper. If your dog has a skin irritation, stop using immediately. Avoid tea tree oil because it is toxic to both cats and dogs.
- Add lemon, which is a natural flea deterrent. Add a cup of lemon juice to your dog's weekly bath, or simply squeeze some onto the comb while you're brushing the dog — to naturally keep the bugs away.

The download kit includes recipes for a natural flea collar and natural bug spray.

5. Dental Care

Dental disease affects many dogs older than the age of four and can lead to serious health problems and complications that go way beyond their mouth. Bacteria can enter the bloodstream and cause problems in the heart, kidneys, and liver. The biggest warning sign is their breath: If it stinks, that's an indication their oral health is suffering.

Dental disease occurs as plaque-forming foods and bacteria build up on your dog's teeth and it hardens into tartar. From there, gingivitis, receding and bleeding gums, and tooth loss are all possible — conditions that are painful to your pup. Prevention is easy: Brushing your dog's teeth is the gold star when it comes to preventing serious periodontal disease.

There are many commercial dog toothpastes on the market. Be sure to look for ones that are natural, organic, and without toxic ingredients. Never use human toothpaste because fluoride can irritate a dog's stomach.

Introduce your pups to tooth brushing slowly. Start by rubbing your finger in a circular motion inside their mouth to get them used to it before you try with a toothbrush. Rewarding with a small treat afterwards also makes the process more palatable!

The American Society for the Prevention of Cruelty to Animals (ASPCA) advises pet owners to wrap a piece of gauze around their index finger and apply canine toothpaste to the tip, or a paste made with baking soda and water. In addition to brushing and chewing, regular scaling treatments in the vet's office will remove all tartar buildup.

5.1 Antlers: An eco-friendly tooth cleaner

Free of preservatives, chemicals, and additives, antlers from animals such as deer and elk make a fantastic natural chew that gives your dog's teeth a great cleaning. As your pup grinds down the antler to get to the marrow inside, the antler gently massages their gums and cracks away plaque and tartar on the teeth. It also contains naturally occurring minerals to aid health such as calcium, potassium, iron, and zinc.

Most antlers sold in pet stores come from wild-roaming animals, where the antler has shed naturally, so it's a humane treat too! Depending on how hard your dog chews, these treats can last for many months, and are ground down to tiny nubs, so there's very little waste. Just make sure to take the treat away when it's too small for them to grip, so they don't swallow the nub. You can find antlers at most major pet retailers or online through Amazon.

6. Playtime, Exercise, and Enrichment

The pet obesity epidemic sweeping North America stems in large part from the fact we are showering our dogs with food and treats rather than what they really need: socialization, playtime, and exercise. A sedentary dog quickly becomes a bored and fat dog, with health and behavioral problems not far behind.

The culprit is our busy lives, and the time we spend in front of screens: The 2011 Canadian Pet Wellness Report found that pet owners spend three times as much time watching TV and nearly twice as much time surfing the Internet than they do playing with and exercising their pets.[11]

Instead of buying your dogs another toy or trinket, find ways to keep them physically and mentally active. There are many great ways to do this without contributing to carbon emissions, including spending time together, hands-on training, participating in sporting classes and competitions, and creating do-it-yourself enrichment activities.

Whether it's taking your dog to a park or beach or going on a hike, you are building a bond with your pup without spending money or buying

---

11 "Canada's Pet Wellness Report," Canadian Veterinary Medical Association and Science Diet, accessed January 2016. canadianveterinarians.net/documents/canada-s-pet-wellness-report2011

products that will end up in a landfill. Outdoor adventure time will help your dog live a long and healthy life while also enhancing your own physical and mental well-being.

Certified dog trainer and Vetstreet.com author Mikkel Becker says beyond participating in formal classes for nose work and agility, you can also invigorate your dog's mind by just adding obstacles and challenges into its day.

"Hiding toys inside of a cardboard box for the dog to find or creating a makeshift agility course with things like brooms, cans, chairs, and blankets creates a fun challenge with things you already have," Becker says.

Raid your garage and backyard shed for items to make your own agility course. Weave poles can be created using recycled ski poles and jumps are as simple as balancing thin plywood boards on top of old bricks or cinderblocks.

6.1 Toy time

Owners spend an average of $47 on toys for their dog each year, according to the 2015 to 2016 American Pet Product Association National Pet Owners Survey. This equates to tens of millions of dollars shelled out on toys, many of which are plastic and flimsy, that end up suffering three fates: Being ripped apart by an overzealous pooch, forgotten about, or dumped in the trash after they are destroyed. There are eco-friendly solutions when it comes to playtime — and the toys that come with it.

Investing in a high-quality indestructible toy for Fido eliminates waste. Even if it is made from a nonrenewable material, it is still an eco-friendly option because it will last many years and won't have to be replaced time and time again with new items.

KONG toys, available at major pet retailers, are made from rubber in a variety of sizes and provide dogs with a healthy outlet for chewing and licking, starting from when they are puppies. If stuffed with food, applesauce, or peanut butter, they can be a mentally stimulating treat during crate-training or while trying to curb separation anxiety. They can also be filled with broth and frozen to provide hours of mental stimulation while dogs lick their "pupsicle."

As mentioned in Chapter 1, a recent innovation is the use of recycled plastic water bottles in dog toys. The bottles are cleaned and striped of labels before being chopped into flakes, liquefied, and reengineered into a 100 percent nontoxic, sustainable, and recycled material used to stuff doggie beds and stuffed toys.

There are easy ways to reuse your dog's existing toys or create new ones with items already in your home:

- **Stuffie hospital:** Trainer Mikkel Becker suggests sewing destroyed stuffed animals in a "toy infirmary" so your dog can relive the glory of ripping it apart.

- **Recycle kids toys:** As long as they don't have small pieces or movable parts, unwanted stuffed animals can be handed down to your four-legged family member.

- **Food puzzles:** Use paper towel or toilet paper rolls, old bowls, water bottles, and muffin tins to create a food-based reward puzzle for your dog. Hide several treats inside.

- **Fabric chew toys:** Braid unwanted fabrics into a sturdy tug toy using old T-shirts or socks.

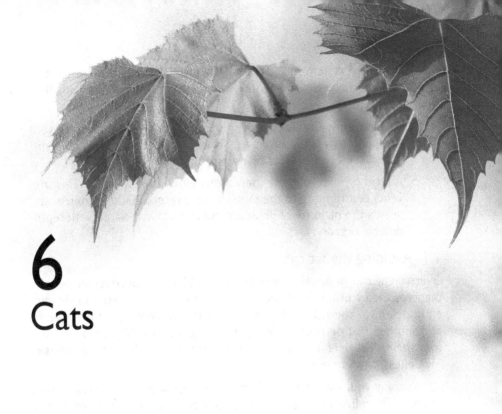

6
Cats

The 2016 survey of the American Pet Products Association estimates there are just shy of 86 million pet cats in the US alone.[1] Now multiply that number by the amount of canned food, bags of kitty litter, toys, and vet trips required for each of those cats … *every* single year. That's a big eco-paw print.

There are ways to lower your cat's impact on the environment but they need to be introduced slowly to guarantee success. Some felines can be notoriously fussy when it comes to smell, taste, and texture, whether that's food or kitty litter, and they don't always take well to sweeping changes.

1. Health and Wellness

The greenest thing you can do for your cat's health is to be proactive about it. Regular veterinary visits will arm you with the tools to keep your cat healthy and catch potential illnesses early, which translates to better outcomes.

Dr. Bruce G. Kornreich, Associate Director of the Cornell Feline Health Center at Cornell University, equates preventative care to the difference between a "health care system" and a "sick care system" for felines.

---

1 "Pets by the Numbers," The Human Society of the United States, accessed January 2016. humanesociety. org/issues/pet_overpopulation/facts/pet_ownership_statistics.html?referrer=https://www.google.ca

"A sick care system means we'll wait for sickness and then treat it. Ethically, financially, environmentally, it's better to maintain health than treat sickness," he says.

- **Vaccinations:** Cradle-to-grave environmental cat care starts with vaccinations at a young age, which eliminates preventative diseases. See Chapter 4 for more information.
- **Altering:** Have your cat spayed or neutered as a kitten. This prevents contributing to the massive pet overpopulation problem and avoids the majority of illnesses and cancers associated with reproductive organs.

1.1 Avoiding the fat cat

Overweight cats suffer the same health problems as overweight people: diabetes, heart problems, hypertension, joint issues, osteoarthritis, and early death. In the US, 29.8 percent of cats are considered overweight and another 28.1 percent are obese, meaning they are 30 percent or more over their ideal weight, according to the most recent National Pet Obesity Awareness Day Survey.[2]

Keeping your cats lean and fit is the kindest and most conscious step to ensure they live a long and healthy life free of diseases and health conditions that are largely preventable. Ask your vet to assess your cat's body condition score during check-ups to determine if it could benefit from shedding a few pounds.

Because cats won't go on a jog the way a dog will, shedding weight is less about exercise and more about disciplined diets. Reduce treats, avoid having kibble available 24/7, follow manufacturer instructions, and provide a food that is high quality and appropriate to your cat's life stage.

1.2 Flea and tick control

Cats allowed outdoors have an increased risk of contracting fleas and ticks, but indoor cats don't live inside a protective bubble, says veterinarian Dr. Cathy Lund of the American Association of Feline Practitioners.

"People and other pets can bring in 'hitchhiker' fleas, and ticks are just as happy to bite a person as they are to bite one of our pets," she says.

Insecticide-based flea and tick control products can protect cats from parasitic infestations and diseases; unfortunately, some chemical products carry potential health risks. To reduce the risk, only use parasite products specifically designed for cats — many products for dogs are a much stronger dose and contain permethrins, which are potentially fatal for cats.

2 "2014 Obesity Facts & Risks," Association for Pet Obesity Prevention, accessed January 2016. petobesity-prevention.org/pet-obesity-fact-risks

"Cats are not small dogs. Those little cat livers cannot detoxify like other species can, and they easily suffer chronic or acute poisoning," says Dr. Nicky Joosting of the Vancouver Feline Veterinary Housecall Service.

There's also an ingestion risk for topical treatments if cats are able to lick off what you've applied. Dr. Lund recommends applying so-called "spot on" products to the base of the skull instead of the shoulder blades, where they can reach with their tongue. Consult with your vet about which product is right for your cat. The download kit includes natural flea and bug remedies for your cat.

1.3 Natural solution to hairballs

Hairballs are caused when cats groom themselves and swallow the hair, which then forms a lump in the digestive tract. This often ends in vomiting. The good news is that you can prevent the majority of hairballs by regular grooming and brushing, especially for cats with longer hair. You can also add a teaspoon of natural food oil (e.g., olive oil) to your cats' food once a week to help lubricate their digestive tract so the hairballs don't create an obstruction.

2. The Problem with Poop

Our tiny feline friends have a big problem: Their poop. They leave about 1.2 million metric tons of it in the environment annually in the US, according to the journal *Parasitology*.[3] Improperly disposed of feces can contaminate waterways, which harms fish, wildlife, and human drinking water. The parasite Toxoplasma gondii in cat poop is harmful to human health, especially pregnant women and those with compromised immune systems. You can greatly reduce environmental harm by always cleaning up after your cat and training it to use a litter box.

Not all municipalities agree on the least harmful way to dispose of cat poop. Many cities are fine with it being flushed down the toilet, where it will eventually be treated at a wastewater facility. However, other regions say it should be thrown in the trash instead, because wastewater facilities may not be able to kill the parasite Toxoplasma gondii if poop is flushed.

Cat feces are not recommended for garden composting because of the parasites and bacteria that could be passed on to people.

2.1 Eco-friendly litter

With rows of different choices at the pet store, it may be hard to believe that kitty litter is actually a relatively new product. The first clay litter was developed in 1947, and many modern brands still use clay. It's cheap and works well, but the strip mining used to produce it is extremely harmful to the environment — and used litter ends up in the landfill.

3 "Toxoplasma Oocysts As a Public Health Problem," E. Fuller Torrey, Robert H. Yolken, Trends in Parasitology, accessed January 2016. cell.com/trends/parasitology/abstract/S1471-4922(13)00090-1

It isn't just harmful to the earth. The quartz silica dust in clay kitty litter can cause respiratory problems in felines, and even asthma. Synthetic perfumes meant to make litter smell better can irritate cats' eyes and aggravate their allergies. Some cats may also be sensitive to pine, wheat, or cedar-based litters.

Opt for a litter that is biodegradable and made from recycled materials. Some brands, such as World's Best Cat Litter, uses recycled corncobs, while Yesterday's News is sourced from postconsumer nontoxic recycled newspaper. There are also eco-friendly litters made from recycled wood fiber pellets, wheat, corn, soy, and tree nut husks (e.g., walnut).

Some cats are notoriously picky about their litter, so introducing them to an eco-friendly litter must be gradual, says veterinarian Dr. Ilona Rodan of the American Association of Feline Practitioners.

"Add in small amounts to the regular litter you are using. We need to make sure the cat likes it so they do not start house-soiling," says Dr. Rodan.

Scooping frequently will reduce the smell of your litter box, and baking soda sprinkled inside makes a natural deodorizer. To reduce waste, avoid purchasing litter box liners.

2.2 How to dispose of kitty litter

There's no getting around it, clay, silica, and crystal litters must be thrown in the trash, which is another reason they're not the best option.

Don't flush litter, even if it's labeled "flushable," because it can clog drains and cause other problems in your personal or municipal septic system.

Biodegradable litters can be composted along with yard waste, but should not be used on any gardens where food is being produced. Stick to ornamental gardens, flowers, and shrubs. Some may be used as mulch or garden fertilizer. Depending on your municipality, you may be able to put the litter out for collection along with your yard trimmings.

3. Indoor versus Outdoor Cats

Outdoor cats get more exercise, stimulation, and natural enrichment than their indoor counterparts, but they are also exposed to a laundry list of dangers: traffic, poisoning, extreme heat and cold, being lost or stolen, disease transmission, parasites, cat fights, and animal attacks. Outdoor cats, on average, live much shorter lives than those that live exclusively indoors.

Besides the harm they're exposed to, free-roaming cats are responsible for huge environmental damage. A 2013 paper from Nature Communications found that outdoor cats are the single biggest killer of birds and small mammals in the US. The numbers are staggering: It estimates cats kill upwards of 4 billion birds and 22.3 billion mammals annually.[4] Cat feces left on lawns and in parks can leach into the ground and contaminate water sources with parasites.

There are ways to give your cats an outdoor experience when they are inside your home:

- **Cat shelves and perches:** Perches and cat "hangouts" installed near a sunny window let your kitty sunbathe and enjoy nature without being in harm's way. These can be purchased in pet stores or you can easily make your own.

- **Bird TV:** Hang a bird feeder or bird bath outside a window where your cat can easily view it. Make sure the window is tightly secured and your cat has a comfy spot to sit. This "Bird TV" will provide hours of entertainment.

3.1 Safe outdoor time: Leash walking and catios

A good compromise is giving your cats access to the outdoors in a protected way that does not put their health or the environment at risk. With patience and rewards, cats can be trained to walk on a leash. Starting at a young age increases the likelihood of success.

If you have a yard, consider building a protected cat patio — or "catio" — to give your indoor cat an outdoor experience. These fenced-in outdoor enclosures allow access to sunshine, fresh air, sounds, stimulation, and nature while keeping winged creatures safe from predation. You can construct perches to let your kitty lounge in the sun and shelves to climb.

The construction can be eco-friendly and doesn't have to cost a lot of money. You can build your catio with upcycled boards from other projects, and wire mesh or chicken wire to keep your cat secure. Pinterest is full of catio ideas for every design, budget, and style.

4. Natural Alternatives to Declawing

For many decades an acceptable way to discourage the very natural behavior of scratching was to perform a very unnatural surgery: declawing. The tidal wave of public opinion is changing on this controversial procedure, which actually amputates a cat's claw at the last toe joint.

Veterinary associations in North America now agree the procedure can cause long-term negative health effects — and say it is a poor substitute for finding solutions to problem scratching.

---

4 "The Impact of Free-Ranging Domestic Cats on Wildlife of the United States," Scott R. Loss, Tom Will, and Peter P. Marra, Nature Communications, accessed January 2016. nature.com/ncomms/journal/v4/n1/full/ncomms2380.html

4.1 The four Rs of appropriate scratching

It may seem like your cats are purposefully trying to destroy your living room with their scratching, but that's not the motivation behind this instinctual behavior. Scratching is a form of kitty communication, letting them mark their territory visually and through scent, as the outer layer of their claws are shed as they scratch. It's also entertaining and lets them get a good stretch. Use the following four Rs to naturally minimize damage and create appropriate scratching opportunities:

- **Reduce the damage:** Regular claw trimmings will minimize damage to furniture when scratching occurs. You can also purchase temporary, nontoxic vinyl kitty nail caps that are glued to your cat's nails that protect against destruction.

- **Repel:** Does kitty have a favorite couch to destroy? Cover any areas you don't want scratched with unappealing textures, such as tinfoil or double-sided tape. A natural pheromone spray, such as Feliway, sprayed onto the area can reduce a cat's desire to scratch there again.

- **Redirect and reward:** Provide multiple appropriate scratching posts and reward heavily when they use them. You can even rub a bit of catnip on the new post to add some enticement.

Skip the store bought scratching posts and make your own. The Internet is full of blueprints for DIY eco-friendly posts. Source natural materials such as sisal, rope, discarded wood, old carpet, and recycled cardboard to create scratching outlets that are tailored to your cat's preferences.

5. Playtime: The Cat's Meow

Cat play is much more than just fun. It provides mental and physical stimulation to ward off lethargy, depression, and weight issues. It also allows cats to express natural behaviors such as hunting, climbing, jumping, hiding, and pouncing. Playing is also a natural way to increase the human-cat bond.

If you've ever seen a cat play in an empty cardboard box, you know you don't need to spend a lot of money to keep your cat entertained. Here are some ideas for eco-friendly toys made from items around your home — and play ideas that don't contribute to the landfill:

- **Hiding/investigating:** Empty boxes and paper shopping bags with the handles removed make fantastic structures to investigate and play in. Cut out windows and doors in a large cardboard box to make a kitty palace to explore.

- **Give old items new life:** A crumpled piece of brown paper or paper towel roll can become something to chase. Wine corks, old ping-pong balls, and even pen lids are great for batting and chasing.

- **Predator play:** Let your cat act out its prey instinct with toys designed to imitate hunting. String a felt toy or feather at the end of a rod and wave it to mimic a bird in flight. Let your cat "catch" the prey. Stuff a small felt toy with organic catnip and let them chase and catch it.

- **Source sustainable:** If you're buying cat toys, look for items made from recycled goods or sustainable materials, such as sisal and hemp. Avoid plastics. Buy from local companies that make their products nearby.

- **Swap toys:** Cats can become bored with their toys but that doesn't mean you need to constantly buy new ones. To make old toys magically new again, remove half of your cat's toys and rotate in new ones every few weeks.

- **Companion kitty:** Instead of you doing all the entertaining, why not let a companion kitty do it for you? Groups such as Vancouver Orphan Kitten Rescue Association recommend adopting kittens in pairs because they will entertain each other and burn off energy together.

6. Cat Food

With a dizzying selection of kibbles, canned, raw, and freeze-dried foods sold in pet stores, it's nearly impossible to decipher which are the most nutritious, let alone eco-friendly and sustainable.

Being green starts with the food packaging itself. Always recycle cat food tins, and look for pouches that are made from non-BPA plastic that can be recycled. The following are some strategies to lower the carbon footprint associated with your feline friends.

6.1 Decoding labels

Marketers try to lure you into buying cat food with packaging displaying wild salmon fillets, T-bone steaks, and whole chicken breasts, but that's not necessarily what's inside.

Whether it's kibble, freeze-dried, canned, or pouches, the quality of meat used for cat food varies wildly and routinely includes rendered by-products from factory farming, meat trimmings, and even so-called 4D animals (i.e., dead, diseased, dying, disfigured), which are all deemed unfit for human consumption. In some cases, after animal protein is cooked down through a rendering process, artificial flavors, colors, preservatives, chemicals, and cheap fillers can be added before it hits store shelves.

"There is a world of difference between quality organic meat proteins and less refined filler agents," says Dr. Cathy Lund. "It is important to research the companies that produce the foods your cat will be eating because not all are created equal."

Unfortunately, a higher price point isn't always an indicator of quality so knowing how to read the food label will go a long way. The following are the legal labeling standards from the Association of American Feed Control Officials (AAFCO):[5]

- **Premium, super premium, holistic:** Buzzword alert! These terms have no legal definition and do not speak to the nutrition or quality of the product.

- **Complete and balanced:** Meets the AAFCO standard for "nutritional adequacy" and can be fed daily. Not an indicator of food quality.

- **Natural:** Generally speaking, this means food that does not contain artificial and chemical additives, preservatives, and colors.

- **Organic:** Produced through methods that promote ecological balance and conserve biodiversity. May not legally contain synthetic fertilizers, sewage sludge, irradiation, and genetic engineering. Must display a US Department of Agriculture (USDA) organic label and contain at least 95 percent organic ingredients.

- **Meat:** Primarily animal flesh but can also include less appealing cuts of meat, such as the heart. Bones are not allowed to be added. The "meat" can come from cows, pigs, sheep, or goats, but it must be identified if it comes from another animal, such as buffalo, fish, or chicken.

- **Meat and animal by-products:** Rendered meat deemed unfit for human consumption, either for aesthetic reasons or because it is parts of the animal people would not eat. That includes lungs, udders, brain, blood, spleen, bones, and intestines. The species of animal must be listed unless it is from cattle, pigs, sheep, or goats.

- **Meat and bone meal:** Highly processed by-product that can contain organ meat, trimmings, and bones. Can also include so-called "4D" animals.

There is no single food that is the best for every cat, so consult with your veterinarian or a feline nutrition specialist to seek the best diet plan for your pet's weight, life stage, activity level, and age.

In general, look for the following:

- Minimally processed

- Organic

- Natural — without preservatives, artificial colors, and flavors.

5 "Reading Labels," Association of American Feed Control Officials (AAFCO), accessed January 2016. talkspetfood.aafco.org/readinglabels

- Made with hormone and antibiotic-free meat, grass fed, and free-range proteins.
- Vegetables sourced from local farms.
- Contains no GMO corn and vegetable crops.
- Does not list "meat and bone meal."

6.2 Ditch the beef and lamb

Cats are obligate carnivores and require nutrients found in meat, including taurine, and vitamins A and B12. Pound for pound, they eat more meat than dogs do, and with that animal protein-heavy diet unfortunately comes greenhouse gas emissions.

Lamb and beef production use the most water and land per pound of any animal protein so opt for meats that are less carbon-belching. Salmon, chicken, turkey, and tuna produce far fewer greenhouse gases, according to the Environmental Working Group.[6] Search for sustainably produced meat and seafood whenever possible.

6.3 Feeding to stay lean and trim

Overweight and obese cats die up to two-and-a-half years earlier than their regular-sized counterparts and require more medications and costly medical interventions, according to the Association for Pet Obesity Prevention (APOP).

From an environmental standpoint, the greenest diet you can give your cats is one that keeps them in a healthy body condition from kitten to senior. Even two extra pounds on your cats greatly increases their risk of debilitating but largely preventable weight-related conditions, including heart and respiratory diseases, kidney disease, and many forms of cancer.

If you have a fat cat, talk to your vet about a weight-loss plan to reduce calories. A trim cat is a happier cat, and will live a much longer and healthier life.

Here are some tips for "fat cat" prevention:

- Don't feed extra meals or treats. This is wasteful and contributes to obesity.
- Avoid free-choice feeding, or having food available 24/7.
- Divide the daily calories by feeding smaller meals more often.
- Don't use an automatic or self-food feeder.
- Follow manufacturer feeding directions.
- Reduce treats: Each small treat can equal 10 percent of daily calories.

---

6 "Meat Eater's Guide: Report," Environmental Working Group, accessed January 2016. ewg.org/meateatersguide/a-meat-eaters-guide-to-climate-change-health-what-you-eat-matters/climate-and-environmental-impacts

- Food isn't love! If your cat is begging at the bowl, give it water or playtime, not more food.

6.4 Age-appropriate food

Just like people, cats have different nutritional requirements depending on their age. Kittens need more protein and calories than adult or sedentary cats, and senior kitties may benefit from a diet with more fatty acids. Selecting a food that is appropriate for your cat's life stage is a healthy choice that ensures its nutritional needs are met.

The Association of American Feed Control Officials (AAFCO), who oversee pet food labeling in the US, provide nutritional adequacy statements on cat food. Avoid buying foods with statements proclaiming the food is "complete and balanced for all life stages" because that may lead to nutritional deficiencies. Instead, look for statements specially mentioning the life stage, including "adult maintenance" and "growth and reproduction."

6.5 Is raw food good for your kitty?

Whether it is for environmental, ethical, nutritional, or humane considerations, many pet parents are shunning traditional pet food and turning to alternative diets for their feline family members. From an environmental standpoint, these diets can have a lower carbon footprint than buying food at the pet store, but the cat's nutritional needs must always be put first.

If you decide to implement a raw, homemade, or vegetarian diet, only do so in consultation with your veterinarian and a feline nutritionist — and monitor the cat's health. Otherwise, your good intentions could be putting your pet's well-being in jeopardy.

Some cat owners believe feeding raw proteins instead of retail pet food more accurately mimics how their predator pets would hunt and eat in the wild. Believers in the raw diet tout a range of health benefits, including shinier coats, healthier teeth and gums, tinier poops, and better weight control.

The diet is greener than conventional food for many reasons:

- Cats on a raw diet produce less biological waste because more of the protein is absorbed into their bodies.
- You can buy meat from local farmers, reducing the carbon footprint of shipping food a great distance.
- You can source organic and "humane" meat, and food with no fillers, artificial ingredients, GMO crops, or chemicals.

Veterinary associations in North America discourage feeding raw meats because they may not be nutritionally complete, and there is a risk of pathogen contamination for both the cat and the humans who come into contact with it. People who choose to feed raw say the concerns are overblown and the risks are easily mitigated with proper food handling.

6.6 DIY pet chef

Concerned over what goes into commercial cat food, some pet owners are opting to make their own meals in a bid to control exactly what goes into their kitty's dinners.

By sourcing your own local meats and vegetables you can ensure a diet free of chemicals, preservatives, and pesticides, and virtually eliminate plastic packaging, not to mention the carbon footprint of transportation.

There are thousands of recipes online to make your own cat food and design meal plans, but you have to do your homework to ensure the meals are properly supplemented with the right vitamins and minerals.

The Cornell Feline Health Center at Cornell University discourages the DIY diet, and says anyone who chooses this option should work with a vet and nutritionist to ensure the cat's dietary needs are being met.

6.7 Can cats go vegetarian?

It's absolutely true that a vegetarian or vegan diet has a smaller carbon footprint — but most vets reject the assertion that these naturally carnivorous animals can thrive on this diet.

Cats require a range of nutrients and vitamins that are found in meat, including taurine, carnitine, B12, and Vitamin D; otherwise, they can suffer serious health issues. Taurine deficiency can lead to eye and heart problems, and even heart failure. That health risk is why vets warn against feeding meatless diets to felines.

If you choose to feed vegetarian, it is crucial that you do your research and meet your cat's nutritional requirements through supplements. Some brands, such as Vegepet, promise all the nutrients that cats require, but they are derived from nonanimal sources. Speak to your vet and a nutritionist before going veggie for your cat.

6.8 Garden of eating: A feline-friendly garden

Growing an indoor supply of cat grass provides your feline friends a safe outlet for grazing and the supplemental greens in their diet also help their digestive tract. This is especially true for indoor cats that wouldn't otherwise have access to natural greenery.

Cat grass is actually a cereal grass similar to oat or wheat that will wilt after several weeks, so plant several pots a few weeks apart for a continuous supply. Planting is easy: Buy seeds from your local garden store and start growing them in potting soil in a sturdy four-inch plant pot. It will take around two weeks for the shoots to germinate and grow. Your cat can enjoy it for a few weeks before you need to pull out the remaining shoots and plant more seeds. Oat grass also works well.

You can also grow a catnip plant and give your cat the leaves fresh, or let them dry. This plant needs to be grown in an outdoor environment. Cats love the natural high they get from this plant.

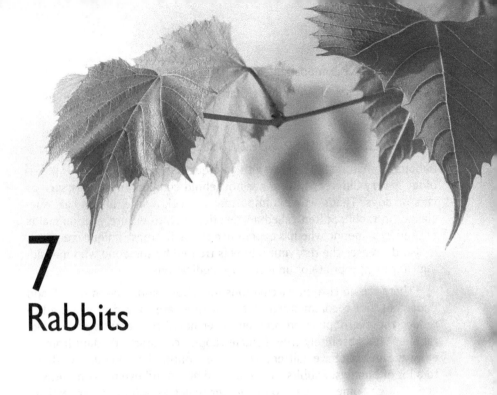

7
Rabbits

Cute, fluffy, and packed with personality, rabbits are often called the ultimate vegan pet because these herbivores shun meats and dairy in favor of munching hay and fresh vegetables. They're also "zero waste" because you can compost their poop to fertilize your garden to produce more veggies to feed them! Sadly, many of these eco-friendly animals end up abandoned or relegated to backyard hutches because they're considered "starter pets" and buyers don't realize they can live for more than a decade. These prey animals love playing on the ground but don't like being held or cuddled, which means they aren't suitable for young children, even though they're often given to kids.

These clean and intelligent animals are highly social and absolutely love having a buddy to play with so consider adopting a pair of bonded bunnies to keep each other company.

Here are the top five reasons rabbits are eco-friendly pets:

- They're herbivores.
- You can grow your own rabbit food.
- Hyper local: You can reduce your carbon footprint by sourcing hay and veggies from area farms.

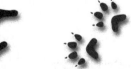

- They have compostable poop.
- Rabbits are clean animals that generally don't require shampoos, tick medications, and drugs.

1. Vet Care: Seek a Specialist

Rabbits are natural herbivores with a unique hindgut system. Their physiology is very different from other household companion animals such as cats or dogs. That's why it's important to seek a veterinarian that specializes in rabbits, often called an "exotics" vet, to ensure your animal is treated by someone who has experience caring for these unique creatures. It also decreases the risk your bunny is treated by someone who may administer inappropriate or unnecessary medications.

There are no current vaccinations for rabbits approved in the US and Canada but it's recommended that both sexes are spayed or neutered to reduce the overpopulation problem. Ever heard the term "breeding like rabbits"? It's absolutely true: Female rabbits can start breeding from an early age and can have a litter *every* single month. That can quickly add up to a lot of bunnies. Rabbits can be altered at around five to six months of age, though some rescue groups neuter males as soon as their testicles drop (i.e., around nine weeks) to prevent unwanted litters.

Altering your female bunny is also an easy way to avoid common health concerns, such as malignant cancers and uterine diseases. Neutered males will exhibit less negative behaviors, such as marking their territory and nipping at other rabbits, or their owners.

1.1 How to find a rabbit-friendly vet

Veterinarians that specialize in rabbits can be harder to find and more expensive than a traditional vet. To find one, start by asking your local animal shelter or rescue or use the Internet to search "exotic vets" in your area.

The House Rabbit Society (rabbit.org/vet-listings) and Association of Exotic Mammals Veterinarians (aemv.org) provide online lists of veterinarians in North America and abroad that specialize in medicine on rabbits.

1.2 Teeth that keep growing

Unlike humans, the teeth of rabbits grow continuously throughout their life. They can grow into painful needle-like points that will need to be clipped or filed by a vet if they're not worn down naturally. The number one way to ensure your rabbit's teeth grind down appropriately is to provide unlimited or "free choice" grass-based hays to chew.

"When a rabbit chews it has a horizontal movement in the back of their mouth, and grinding the hay has a larger movement than if they were just being fed grains and pellets," says Dr. Peter G. Fisher, owner of Pet Care Veterinary Hospital and past president of the Association of Exotic Mammal Veterinarians.

Providing free-choice hay will also decrease the likelihood of painful gastrointestinal blockages that can make rabbits sick. Rabbits can end up with intestinal slowdowns from ingesting wads of hair when they are grooming themselves, because they can't throw up or hack up a hairball like cats can.

Rabbits are prey animals and they'll hide symptoms of sickness and pain — sometimes for years — so they don't appear vulnerable. A warning sign that a rabbit is sick is that it is not eating and can't be tempted with fruit or other high-reward treats, says Lisa Hutcheon, Co-Founder of Small Animal Rescue Society of BC. Teeth problems and gut blockages can be painful and may cause a rabbit to stop eating — and eventually starve.

"They don't have any warning signs the way dogs and cats do. They won't whimper if they have a broken leg," says Hutcheon. "Look in their litter box. If there's no poop, you need to get them to the vet right away."

2. Rabbit Food

Similar to horses, rabbits have what's called a hindgut fermentation system that allows them to break down high-fiber hay and vegetables, which makes up the bulk of their diet.

Protein, fats, and simple carbohydrates are digested in the stomach and small intestine whereas fiber is moved quickly into a sac called the cecum, where it is fermented. Large particles of fiber are pooped out in the form of hard round fecal pellets whereas the contents of cecum are eliminated in the form of soft mucous covered pellets called cecotropes that rabbits quickly re-ingest directly from their anus. It may sound strange, but this is an important part of the rabbit's digestive process!

The cornerstone of every rabbit's diet is grass-based hay, which will keep its teeth worn down and maintain intestinal smoothness. It should compose 70 to 80 percent of its daily diet and should always be available.

Timothy hay is the most common, but other grass-based hays, such as oat hay, brome, or organic meadow grass can be substituted for variety. Legume-based hay, such as alfalfa may be good for a treat, but it contains extra calcium and protein — and more calories — so it should only be given in moderation.

Rabbit Diet Basics

Think about your rabbit's diet like a pyramid. On the bottom is grass-based hay, which should be available to nibble on 24/7. Next comes fresh vegetables, pellets, and finally, small amounts of fruit.

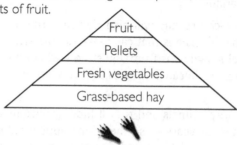

2.1 Rabbit-approved veggies and fruits

Despite a certain unnamed cartoon rabbit constantly munching carrots, these animals actually thrive on a diet of leafy vegetables. They're packed with nutrients and it's nice to give a little variety in taste and texture. Try the following:

- Romaine lettuce
- Green or red lettuce
- Spinach
- Collard greens
- Kale
- Swiss chard
- Mustard greens
- Bok choy
- Herbs such as parsley, cilantro, basil, and mint

Rabbits also love non-leafy and root veggies such as broccoli, celery, cabbage, brussels sprouts, and carrots. These should be fed in smaller amounts because of their sugar and starch content, according to the House Rabbit Society, a nonprofit group dedicated to education about rabbit care.[1] Avoid onions, leeks, and chives because they can lead to blood complications.

For optimum nutrition, buy organic veggies whenever possible, and always wash vegetables thoroughly before feeding to remove any pesticide residue.

High in natural sugars, fruits are sort of like "bunny crack": They love it, but it should only be given as a treat in very small quantities. Rabbits love the following fruits:

---

1 "Suggested Vegetables and Fruits for a Rabbit Diet," House Rabbit Society, accessed January 2016. rabbit.org/suggested-vegetables-and-fruits-for-a-rabbit-diet/#

- Bananas
- Oranges
- Tomatoes
- Grapes
- Melons
- Apples
- Plums
- Papayas
- White nectarines
- Blueberries

Tip: Mash pellets with bananas, carrots, and oats and bake into rabbit biscuit treats.

Pits can be toxic to rabbits, as can apple seeds and stems, so ensure you're only feeding the fruit. The House Rabbit Society advises to leave the skin on the fruit but make sure it's washed thoroughly. Remove it if you're worried about chemical residue or pesticides.

2.2 Hop to it: Sourcing fruits and veggies

You can greatly reduce your environmental footprint by being mindful about how you buy fresh rabbit food, including the following:

- Shop in season, to reduce the distance traveled to marketplace.
- Visit a farmers' market to source local produce.
- Always buy organic (no chemical pesticides/insecticides).
- Ask your grocer for plant scraps and tops that would otherwise be discarded.
- Pick dandelion greens from pesticide-free yards.
- Grow your own.

2.3 Farm-to-rabbit: Grow your own rabbit food

The ultimate "green" way to source veggies for your rabbit is to grow them yourself, and you don't need to live on acreage to do it.

Leafy greens such as lettuces, bok choy, and some herbs can easily be grown in raised beds in a yard or in pots on a patio, says Abi Cushman, founder of MyHouseRabbit.com, an online resource for indoor rabbit owners.

Perhaps the easiest of all herbs to grow in your DIY rabbit garden is mint, which is actually a weed that is very hearty and will crowd out other plants. Because of this, it's best to grow them in containers. Dill, rosemary, and oregano are also suited for container gardening in small spaces.

"Even a beginner gardener with limited space can grow foods for rabbits," says Cushman. "If you are really short on time — and gardening commitment — you can grow dandelions in pots or simply pluck them from your yard. Just make sure the yard isn't treated with chemicals."

2.4 Become friends with a farmer

The most eco-friendly way to source hay is from local farms. From an ecological and ethical perspective, buying through this farm-to-rabbit method is great for a number of reasons:

- Avoids large carbon footprint of having products shipped great distances to you.
- Decreased packaging waste. You can bring your own container to transport it.
- Supporting local farmers, which will in turn support your local community.
- Buying in bulk is much more economical. You can buy a 50-pound box online from a commercial source to reduce packaging waste.

You can buy a bale of hay roughly as big as the backseat of your car for $11 to $20, versus paying $9 for a small bag in a pet store, says Lisa Hutcheon of the Small Animal Rescue Society of BC. She recommends storing it in a shed or garage and ensuring it's well aerated to prevent mold.

3. Compost Your Rabbit Poop

Unlike the feces of carnivorous pets such as cats and dogs, which can contain bacteria that make it unsafe to put in your vegetable garden, rabbit poop is 100 percent compostable and is therefore safe to use on gardens that produce food.

Because they are herbivores, hay and veggie-filled rabbit droppings can be added to your compost pile and converted into a fantastic odor-free manure for vegetable plants and your home garden. Some owners will even spread the droppings directly onto the soil. The high nitrogen and phosphorus content of rabbit poop makes it a nutrient-rich and organic fertilizer for both ornamental and veggie gardens.

Starting your own rabbit waste composter is simple. Either purchase a compost bin or just start a pile in your yard or garden. From there you can compost the entire content of your rabbit's litter box: droppings, soiled hay, and even the recycled-paper litter, says Abi Cushman of MyHouseRabbit.com.

"So it's not only easy to clean a rabbit's litter box — by just dumping everything out onto your compost pile — it also greatly reduces the amount of waste going to a landfill," Cushman says. "Add in some tea bags, vegetable scraps, grass clippings, and fallen leaves to your compost and you'll have a great mix."

3.1 Litter box 101

Similar to cats, rabbits can be easily trained to use a litter box. However, using litter designed for cats can harm your rabbit's health and the environment. Here's what you need to know about the products on the market.

You should avoid the following:

- **Clay litters:** These are dusty and can lead to respiratory issues in your rabbit if ingested over time. The deodorants used in these products can be toxic, according to the House Rabbit Society.[2]

- **Pine and other wood-based litters:** Cedar and pine-based litters can emit aromas that can irritate the respiratory system. It can also hurt a rabbit's digestive system if eaten.

- **Clumping cat litters:** Once wet, these litters can stick to your rabbit's fur, which can lead to ingestion after grooming. That's why these litters can cause digestive upset and gastrointestinal blockages. Breathing in the dust causes respiratory issues in some animals.

You may want to try the following:

- **Recycled paper:** Made from recycled newspaper and other postconsumer paper, these litters are lower in dust and less likely to cause respiratory issues. If you decide to use these products, be careful about what the source of that paper is, says Dr. Micah Kohles, Oxbow's Director of Veterinary Science and Outreach and President of the Association of Exotic Mammal Veterinarians. "You want to go with something that is higher quality and not full of inks and chemicals," says Dr. Kohles, adding that it's often difficult to identify what postconsumer materials end up in recycled paper products. Look for recycled products that are produced with paper that used soybased ink.

- **Compressed straw:** These litters are 100 percent natural, with a very small amount of clay to bind the product. They are more absorbent than newspaper-based products, dust-free, and won't irritate the GI tract if accidentally ingested occasionally, says Dr. Kohles. It's biodegradable and can be composted or flushed down the toilet.

4. Indoor Living Equals a Safe, Happy, and Long Life

Rabbits are a prey animal in nature and that's no different when they're out in your yard, where they can become a target for wild animals

---

2 "Litter Training," House Rabbit Society, accessed January 2016. rabbit.org/faq-litter-training-2

such as raccoons and coyotes but also domesticated pets such as cats and dogs. Most veterinary associations and rabbit-rescue advocates agree that rabbits will live a longer and healthier life if they are kept inside and free from dangers, such as the following:

- Predators (e.g., hawks, roaming pets)
- Extreme temperature fluctuations (i.e., dampness and drafts)
- Toxicity from chemical insecticides sprayed on grass
- Escaping the yard by digging
- Picking up parasites

Just like people, rabbits benefit highly from daily exercise outside their cage. Just make sure you bunny-proof your home the way you would with a baby.

Bunnies like chewing on electrical wires so secure and move any computer and TV cables in their path. Dr. Peter G. Fisher says it's common to see rabbits with lead toxicity if they chew on a baseboard in an older home with lead paint. Your best bet for letting your bunnies stretch their legs while keeping them safe? Supervise them.

Supervised outdoor time is also a great physical and mental stimulation for these curious creatures, as long as it's done in a safe way, says Dr. Micah Kohles. Rabbits can roam and graze on your lawn, provided it hasn't been treated with pesticides or insecticides.

"It's great nutritionally and mentally and it's fun for them — but they need to be protected from predators," Dr. Kohles says.

5. DIY Rabbit Toys

In the wild, rabbits are in constant motion, whether it's tracking down food or trying to avoid becoming the dinner of another animal. That's why it's key to give domesticated rabbits toys and enrichment activities to keep them mentally stimulated and entertained.

"They're very interactive, they love social interaction," says Dr. Micah Kohles. "Getting them out of the cage and allowing them to be active as well as stimulating play is really important."

You don't need to head to the pet store because many common household items can be made into great do-it-yourself enrichment toys. Try the following:

- Homemade castles and hiding houses: Rabbits love to hide. Cut entrances into an overturned cardboard box to create a bunny castle.
- Put your old telephone book into your bunny's pen and let it shred it.

- Roll up an old towel with a few treats and let your bunny burrow.
- Stuff toilet paper or paper towel rolls with Timothy hay so they can burrow, dig, and shred.
- Rooting box: Fill an old planter with organic soil to let your rabbit root.
- Digging box: Fill a cardboard box with hay and toys and let them go wild.

If you do buy commercial or pet store toys, look for items made from natural materials that are biodegradable, such as 100 percent Timothy hay braided into different shapes.

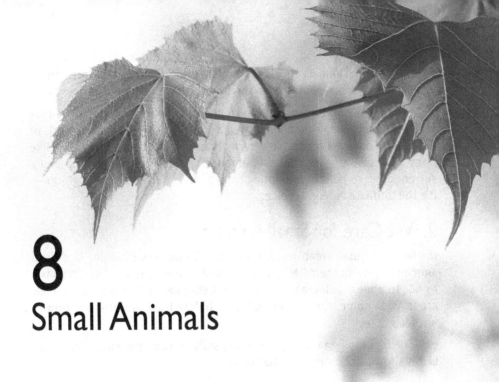

8
Small Animals

This chapter discusses eco-friendly care for mice, rats, hamsters, gerbils, and Guinea pigs. These little guys may be small in body but they're big in personality! With the exception of the Syrian hamster, these wee critters are super social so consider adopting in pairs so they keep each other happy and entertained.

Even though they have a small price tag and are often purchased as starter pets for children, these furry friends still require regular vet visits and responsible, compassionate care. There are also hundreds of dollars in annual costs for food pellets, fresh vegetables, hay and cage litter, and shavings.

Small pets have a much tinier carbon footprint than larger animals such as cats and dogs. They eat less, they poop less, and they live shorter lives. There are simple steps you can take to make sure you're being the most environmentally conscious guardian possible to these so-called "pocket pets."

1. Finding a Little Buddy

Most big-box pet stores source small animals from for-profit commercial enterprises whose goal is to produce the most animals for the lowest cost.

From there, the animals are shipped by truck or plane across North America, adding a carbon footprint to their lives before they're ever bought.

Seek locally bred animals from smaller mom and pop operations that may produce a small number of pets, or work with a local network of breeders. Contact a reputable veterinarian to ask for references. Just like dogs and cats, an overwhelming amount of small animals end up being surrendered, so consider adopting from a local shelter or rescue group — it's the ultimate "green" choice.

2. Vet Care for Small Animals

In the wild, small creatures are prey to all manners of larger birds and animals, so it's in their DNA to always look like they're on their "A game" as not to appear vulnerable — and risk being eaten. When these animals are in your home, they're very good at hiding their symptoms if they're not feeling well.

The biggest sign your pocket pet is suffering and you should call a vet is if it shows any changes in the "three As":

- Appetite
- Activity level
- Attitude

"These are such creatures of habits, so when those habits change it's an indication something is wrong — and the chances are they've been sick for a few weeks," says Dr. Micah Kohles, Oxbow's Director of Veterinary Science and President of the Association of Exotic Mammal Veterinarians.

There are no recommended vaccines for these species but the number one thing you can do to ensure a healthy long life is doing an annual vet exam, where they can be weighed and checked for any underlying health issues.

3. A Balanced Diet

Commercial-pellet feed for Guinea pigs and hamsters; and lab blocks for mice, rats, and gerbils provide a balanced diet of vitamins, minerals, and fatty acids. Seek products that are natural with high-fiber, made from premium ingredients that don't contain artificial ingredients and colors. Thankfully, it won't cost you a lot more to buy a healthy, organic feed free of preservatives and chemicals, says Dr. Micah Kohles.

"Spending an extra $2 or $3 on a bag of food that will last a month will go a long way to get a product that is light years away in terms of nutrition," he says.

The following are what to avoid in kibble, pellets, and lab blocks:

- Animal by-products, including fat, tallow, and bone meal
- Artificial colors, including FD&C reds, yellows, and blues
- Corn syrup and high-fructose corn syrup
- Fillers and preservatives

Guinea pigs in particular should not be fed multicolor pellets and seed mixes because they are what's called a "concentrate selector." This means they'll pick out what's the most appealing, which inevitably means the pellets with artificial sweeteners and colors — the junk food pellets!

3.1 Variety and veggies

Any person would get sick of eating the same meal every day and small animals are no different. Supplement their diet with natural and nutritious food that are appropriate for that species, whether that's fresh grasses, vegetables, or fruits, to mimic what they would eat in the wild.

Guinea pigs need to have Timothy or other grass-based hays available "free choice," which means constantly available in their enclosure. Chewing on this fibrous feed helps them wear down their teeth, which grow continuously throughout their life, and can overgrow and cause severe pain if not ground down naturally. Sourcing hay from a local farm is the most eco-friendly choice, and reduces the packaging and transportation.

Up to 20 percent of the diets of mice, rats, hamsters, and gerbils can be made up of leafy greens, including green and red lettuces, kale, mustard, and collard greens. You can also provide small amounts of fruit, such as apple, melon, and banana, but these high-sugar treats should make up no more than 5 percent of their diet.

To make the greenest choice when it comes to vegetables, choose ones that are locally produced, pesticide-free, organic, and non-GMO. Go to the local farmers' market for farm-to-pet food or, better yet, grow them yourself, says KC Theisen, Director of Pet Care Issues for the Humane Society of the United States (HSUS).

"A great experience for kids is to grow a window box with baby lettuces to use for treats for furry pets," Theisen says. "Animals love an organic, pesticide-free diet as much as we do."

If your small pet is an omnivore, such as a rat or hamster, you can round out their diet with a bit of leftover protein from your own meals, including cooked meats, eggs, plain pasta, and small amounts of dairy.

3.2 Five ways to reduce food waste

Tiny animals only consume tiny food portions, but there are still easy steps you can take to decrease the waste associated with their diet:

- **Don't overfeed:** Use a measuring cup and appropriately sized feeding dishes instead of "eyeballing" portion sizes. This way the animal only eats what it needs and you won't be discarding excess.
- **Divert dinner:** Supplement your pet's food with animal-appropriate items from your own plate.
- **Store food properly:** Keep small animal food in airtight glass containers to seal in freshness. If you use hay, keep it in a dry and well-ventilated area to prevent it from getting moist.
- **Use caution when buying in bulk for small pets:** Bigger bags can go stale in three months. Because pocket pets eat such a small amount, this means you'll end up discarding large volumes of food if it expires.
- **Compost leftovers:** Food, including kibble, hay, nuts, seeds, fruits, and veggies can go in your compost heap to produce great organic fertilizer for your home garden.

3.3 Foraging: Natural health

Grazing on grass helps the health of your Guinea pig — and can trim your lawn in the process! Grass hays are a natural part of the Guinea pig's diet, but letting it munch on fresh grass outside is mentally stimulating, a form of easy entertainment, and adds much-needed vitamin C to its diet. Hamsters also love it.

If you let your pet go outside to forage just ensure that no pesticides and chemical fertilizers have been used on the lawn. Supervision for outdoor foraging is a necessity. Small pets are always in danger of prey animals (e.g., raccoons and hawks), but even family pets such as cats and dogs may enter the yard and cause them harm. Remember: The smaller the pet the higher likelihood of it escaping.

4. Cage Bedding, Litter, and Cleaning

All commercial cage beddings and litters create a carbon footprint during their production. However, there are great compostable and recycled options for small animals that keep them dry, safe, and comfortable and don't contribute to the landfill or hurt their health.

Avoid the following:

- **Pine and cedar shavings or chips:** These soft woods contain aromatics or phenols that can be irritating to the upper gastrointestinal tracts of small animals, especially rats and hamsters.
- **Clumping litters:** Clay-based litters can cause intestinal blockages if ingested, which can occur if your pet grooms itself after using.

- **Reclaimed mill fiber:** Some products made with recycled sawdust from lumber-mill processing appear to be eco-friendly because it's recycled, but some brands can contain nasty chemicals and heavy metals you may not want near your animal or in your home. Do your research before purchasing any of these types of bedding.

Try the following:

- **Eco straw:** These pellets are made with compressed high-fiber wheat straw and are more absorbent than newspaper-based litters. This dust-free litter can be composted or flushed down the toilet.

- **Recycled paper litters:** Litters like Yesterday's News are nontoxic, made from recycled newspaper, and are very absorbent. The packaging is recyclable and the litter is compostable.

- **Recycled newspaper:** You can give your old newspapers a new use by lining the cage with them, and shredding some on top to make a "fluffy" bedding layer, says Elena Kern, President of the United Mouse Club in New York. "Mice like to run through the shreds of paper like it's a game," Kern says, adding that it does have to be cleaned more frequently than other options.

4.1 Cage cleaning

A common cage cleaning ritual goes something like this: Pull dirty litter out and put it into a small plastic bag, then dump it into a plastic trash bag, which eventually goes into a landfill. The problem is that every time you wrap animal waste in another layer of plastic it makes it exponentially more difficult for it to compost and go back into the earth.

The solution is easy: Ditch the plastic. Using paper bags to dispose of litter and animal waste is much more natural and speeds up the process of decomposition. Or look for bags made from compostable and biodegradable materials. Visit Chapter 1 for a full list of great options.

In some municipalities loose litter can be placed in the yard trimmings bin for pick up, as long as it's made from paper, sawdust, corn husks, or wood shavings. Make sure to check with your municipality beforehand.

Home cleaners that use bleaches and other harsh chemicals can cause respiratory damage to small pets. Instead, use an eco-friendly cleaner to clean and wash the cage thoroughly every week.

"If you can smell it, it's time to change the bedding. That's how you treat odor, not by masking it," says Dr. Adrian Walton, from the Dewdney Animal Hospital in Maple Ridge, British Columbia.

Hot water with a drop of nontoxic dish soap and a splash of vinegar works well. The download kit includes recipes for green and safe cleaning agents.

5. Composting Small Animal Poop

While the poop of carnivorous animals such as cats and dogs isn't appropriate to compost because of pathogens, the waste of herbivorous small animals such as Guinea pigs, gerbils, and hamsters is a great addition to your home garden.

You can sprinkle their droppings directly on your garden, but most pet owners prefer to compost it first. The high nitrogen and phosphorus content enriches the soil it's spread into and makes an organic fertilizer for lawns as well as flower and vegetable gardens.

Composting also makes cage cleaning a snap: If you use recycled paper liner or wheat straw bedding, you can also throw that into your compost heap along with their droppings and leftover food.

Some cities prefer small animal poop to be flushed down the toilet where it can be sent to a wastewater plant and treated alongside other sewage. This option ensures the feces won't leach into groundwater, where it can be swept into local waterways and pollute drinking water for humans.

6. A Little Playtime

All small animals benefit greatly from enrichment toys and activities both inside and outside their enclosure. Besides the physical benefits of exercise and play, toys and chewing apparatuses also benefit these intelligent and curious creatures mentally and emotionally.

You can make toys from items you already have in your home, with a low environmental footprint:

- Folded over paper bags and newspapers to create tunnels.
- Paper towel and toilet paper rolls, stuffed with hay and a few treats.
- Cardboard boxes with doors cut out and made into hidey castles and climbing apparatuses.
- Upturned, untreated flower pot to use as separated bedroom space.
- Untreated piece of 4 x 4 wood with holes drilled into it. Stuff holes with hay, cardboard, and treats.
- Natural rope hung from cage for hamsters and mice to use as a swing.
- Plain craft sticks are great for chewing.
- Clean pinecones.
- String a shirt sleeve or sock in your rat's cage to create a sleeping hammock.
- Create a rat nesting box using a Kleenex or cardboard box.

You can also find green solutions at pet stores:

- Branch balls made from natural untreated willow: Perfect for rats, mice, gerbils, and hamsters.
- Untreated branches tied into small bundles.
- Compressed recycled cardboard rings and toys.
- Braided toys made from organic Timothy hay.
- Wooden toys and blocks: Use untreated, uncolored wood.

Many wooden toys in pet stores can be decorated with colored paint that is highly toxic if chewed, so steer clear of those.

6.1 Branching out: Sourcing wood for chewing

Tree branches are an all-natural chew treat for Guinea pigs, hamsters, rats, and mice that provide hours of entertainment while keeping their teeth healthy. They can also be used to create climbing apparatuses in their enclosure.

Many commercial pet stores sell branches and bundles for this purpose, but you can also collect your own, as long as you're careful about which ones you select. The most suitable tree branches for small pets are from fruit trees such as plum, peach, apple, pear, or cherry. Other safe branches include willow, birch, and maple.

Plucking a branch from a random tree carries health risks because you don't know if it has mold, or whether it was treated with pesticides or sprayed for plant rot or mosquitos. So always get it from a known source. Wash any branch you intend on giving to your pet. Your local nursery is also a great source for trimmings and tree cuttings.

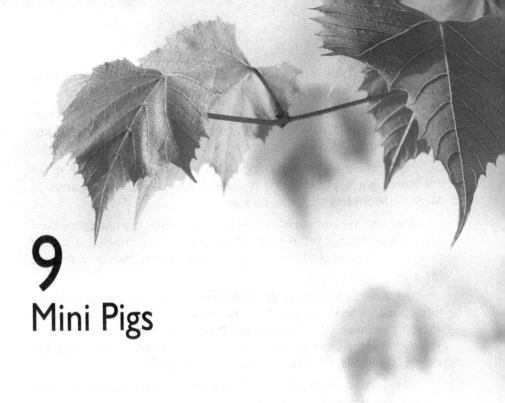

9
Mini Pigs

With intellects rivaling that of a four-year-old child, pigs are charming, easy to train, and have a great personality. It's not hard to see why their popularity as a companion animal has soared in recent years.

Make no mistake though, these complex creatures are no ordinary house pet. They live for 15 years or longer, and their curiosity leads them to become destructive if they're left alone for long periods of time, or not allowed to engage in their natural activities such as foraging and rooting. A bored house pig will rip up carpet, knock over garbage cans, and break into kitchen cupboards, so owners need to pig proof their home the way they would for a baby.

This chapter discusses strategies about how to make sound environmental choices when caring for your little piggy, which is surprisingly easy when it comes to these clean, green pets.

1. Little Pigs, Big Problems: Will They Really Stay Small?

While mini pigs are much smaller than their full-size commercial hog counterparts, which can weigh upwards of 1,000 pounds, they are still

89

much larger than the average dog. Breeders use terms such as "teacup" and "micro" to describe a smaller pig, but those aren't actual breeds.

"Micro, micro mini, pocket pig, pixie pig, are all labels used in marketing that have no real connection to the predicted adult size of the pig," says Kimberly Chronister, Vice President of the American Mini Pig Association.

Just as there are different dog breeds, there are 18 or more different breeds of mini pig, including potbellied, Juliana, Göttingen, Kunekune, Meishan, Minnesota Mini, and Yucatan.

When you see a photo of an adorable "micro pig" in a teacup it's likely still a piglet and has yet to grow. Whereas dogs stop growing at around two years of age, pigs continue to grow and add body mass until they are five years old.

Even though a newborn piglet weighs only one or two pounds, it's rare to see an adult pig less than 50 pounds — and most will end up weighing between 80 to 200 pounds! Piggies are also dense creatures: A 100-pound potbellied pig can be the same physical size as a small dog that weighs 35 pounds, says Brandy Street of the BC SPCA.

"At full grown, a 'miniature' potbellied pig can weigh up to 250 pounds and not be overweight," says Street.

2. Zoning Considerations

No matter the size, owning pigs is illegal in many areas because they are considered farm animals or livestock. Despite mini pigs being a fraction of the size of their farm hog cousins, many bylaws still don't differentiate between them.

Before you bring home a pig, contact your local city hall for the official civic regulations. Get them in writing! It's worth noting that some people have successfully lobbied to have laws changed in their town, but you don't want to leave that matter to chance.

While many mini pigs are happy being with you inside the home, they absolutely need an outdoor space to indulge in their natural activities, such as wallowing and rooting. For that reason, pigs aren't suitable pets for apartments and condos, especially if you live in a high-rise where there is an elevator.

Most pet tenancy agreements only include cats and dogs so if you're a renter, make sure to get written permission before adopting one. Many breeders recommend against renters purchasing a pig because they may end up with a new landlord that isn't as supportive of having a swine on the property if their living situation changes.

3. Ethical adoption

The mini-pig industry is largely unregulated in North America. As a result, there are no legal standards for breeders when it comes to breeding practices, the health of their stock, the size they promise their pigs to be, or the conditions where they're raised.

If you're looking to adopt from a breeder, the American Mini Pig Association recommends getting references and asking questions, such as:

- How old are the parents? (If younger than five, they will not show growth potential of offspring. Even if they are older than five, it's worth asking how big the parents are, although that does not guarantee the offspring will be the same size!)
- Will you take the pig back in the event my family can't care for it?
- What veterinary care or certificates do you provide?

The greenest choice you can make for adoption is bringing a pre-owned pig into your home instead of a piglet. The North American Potbellied Pig Association estimates that the gross majority of pigs adopted in the United States — 90 percent — end up being unloaded at a rescue or sanctuary, so there is no shortage of great adoptable piggies![1]

The American Mini Pig Association has an online directory of breeders and rescues it considers ethical and responsible on its website (american-minipigassociation.com).

4. Green Food Choices

Obesity is the number one health concern for pigs and can shave years off their life. Little piggies are grazers and will eat absolutely everything you give them and as a result can become portly porkers in a hurry! Overweight pigs suffer the same health issues as overweight people: joint pain, arthritis, high blood pressure, low energy levels, and respiratory issues.

Think of proper pig nutrition as eco-friendly preventative medicine. Making solid decisions about their diet when they're young will ensure they live healthy, long lives with less trips to the vet. This is the greenest pig care you can give these omnivores.

Instead of treating your pet pigs as a garbage disposal to gobble up leftovers and table scraps, feed them a complete and healthy diet. That includes grains, high-quality organic pig chow, grass, vegetables, and the occasional bits of fruit. The easiest way to lower your pigs' environmental hoof print is giving them a healthy vegetarian diet that's high in fiber. Grazing on grass, hay, bugs, and grubs is a natural way to allow your pet piggies to express their inner omnivore without making an environmental footprint.

---

1 "Pet Porkers Pack Rescues as Trendy Teacup Pigs Fatten Up," Sue Manning, accessed January 2016. bigstory. ap.org/article/4ecae10b200a4135a4a38ec819f2862c/pet-porkers-pack-rescues-trendy-teacup-pigs-fatten

4.1 Best veggies and fruit for piggies

You know the old saying "an apple a day keeps the doctor away"? Well, the swine equivalent is "a salad a day keeps obesity at bay." Greens and vegetables should be a staple in your pig's diet because they help its digestive tract move smoothly and prevent constipation, which happens when it doesn't get enough roughage. Fruit is also great, but should be given only as a treat because of its high-sugar content.

The following are the suggested foods for a pig:

- **Veggies:** Dark leafy greens, some types of lettuces, mustard and collard greens, romaine, kale, squashes, pumpkin, yams, cucumbers, green beans, carrots, celery, broccoli
  - **Avoid:** Spinach and iceberg lettuce
- **Fruits:** Bananas, including peels; apples, including cores; pears; watermelon on the rind
- **Proteins:** Cooked organic beans including pinto, black, and kidney
- **Treats:** Organic cheerios, puffed wheat, dehydrated fruits and veggies, unsalted popcorn
  - **Avoid:** High-fat, high-sugar, and high-salt treats, such as chips, candy, and chocolate

Go "green" with your pig's food:

- Source local. Go to farmers' markets and ask for any beet or carrot tops that would otherwise be discarded. These veggie by-products are great for pigs and still packed with nutrients.
- Shop in season. This minimizes the carbon emissions of food traveling long distances to reach the market. Avoid tinned produce. Freeze fresh fruits and veggies in reusable containers to use when needed.
- Grow your own. Kale, chards, and lettuces are super easy to grow and, depending on your climate, will thrive through most growing seasons.
- Go organic and GMO-free when you can.
- Divert food waste. Ask your local grocer for any "tired" or "ugly" fruits and vegetables being removed from the shelves. Grocery stores will often pitch perfectly good produce because of how it looks, but it still has great nutritional value.

4.2 Grazing and foraging

Grazing and foraging can be considered eco-friendly lawn care. Because the pigs will be eating the grass, make sure they're only allowed access to areas that haven't been treated with insecticides and pesticides. Letting your pet pig forage on your lawn —

- satisfies natural grazing instincts,
- supplements diet with greens and minerals, and
- trims your lawn.

Pigs love exploring the outdoors and rooting, so fence off any vegetable and ornamental gardens you don't want destroyed. Instead, set aside an area in your yard with soft mulch to encourage this natural behavior, including digging out grubs and worms. You can also turn grazing time into playtime by throwing food onto the lawn and letting them root for it.

Outdoor time should be supervised if the area is not secure. Pigs are prey animals and are at risk of a host of predators including wolves, foxes, snakes, hawks, and even pets such as cats and dogs.

Pigs with light or pink skin can get burned the same way as a human with fair skin and need protection from the sun. Make sure there's an accessible shady area and if you don't have a mud pit for them to wallow in — also known as "nature's sunscreen" — you'll have to apply sunscreen.

5. Waste Not: Pig Poop

The biggest way to lower your pig's carbon footprint has nothing to do with what you put in its mouth — it's how you treat what comes out of its rear end. Training your pig to relieve itself outside is the most environmentally friendly option because it means you can avoid using litters in your home, which will likely end up in the landfill.

Most mini pigs are easier to housebreak than a puppy. Contrary to the myth that pigs are messy, these intelligent animals are very clean and prefer to use the same corner to relieve themselves, as far away from their bed as possible.

If you choose to train your piglet to initially use a litter box, some litters are better than others when it comes to their environmental impact and the animal's health.

What to use:

- **Recycled newspaper:** This is the greenest option because you can reuse what you have in your home, and recycle the paper after you dispose of the poop.
- **Compressed natural recycled newspaper pellets:** Commercial brands like Yesterday's News are tough on odors, nontoxic, and made from postconsumer materials.

- **Natural pine shavings or pellets:** These products use 100 percent natural pine reclaimed from lumber mills. They are absorbent and free of synthetic perfumes and chemicals. Most are biodegradable and can be recycled and used for mulch.

What to avoid — the three Cs:

- **Clumping clay cat litter:** Can cause intestinal or bowel blockages if ingested.
- **Corncob litter:** Can cause obstructions if eaten.
- **Cedar shavings:** The aroma and natural oils can cause irritation.

5.1 Disposing pig poop

The issue of how to dispose of pig waste is a tricky one. Most municipalities, who view mini pigs as livestock, don't want it flushed down the toilet or thrown away with the trash. Improperly disposed of pig waste can also end up being washed into local waterways, which can negatively impact drinking water and wildlife that use it.

The good news is you can put this nutrient-rich "black gold" into action to enrich your home garden, and can in turn produce great organic fruits and veggies to feed your family and pig. If your pet is fed a vegetarian diet, the compost is safe to use on food plants. Unlike "hotter" types of manure (i.e., horse or cow), fresh pig waste can be put directly onto plants without burning them.

Nancy Shepherd, author of *Potbellied Pig Parenting*, collects the poop from her 11 pigs in a five-gallon bucket and when it is full, puts it directly onto her garden.

"The poop is amazing," she says. "Since my pigs are vegetarians, their poop has very little odor."

If you prefer to compost the manure before use there are two simple methods: Either start a simple manure pile or build your own pig waste digester (see the download kit for how to make a waste digester).

DIY manure pile: Designate an outdoor area for the pig poop, and layer with yard trimmings, fallen leaves, and even organic kitchen scraps. You can occasionally add garden soil to speed up the process. Turn the pile every few weeks with a pitchfork or shovel. After several months the pig poop will be decomposed and you can use this organic manure in your garden.

Don't be surprised if you see new plants emerging from your manure pile. If you are feeding fruits and vegetables with seeds, some undigested seeds in the poop will start growing new plants in the topsoil.

6. Bored Pig Equals Bad Pig

Pigs are super social and become very bonded to their human family, even suffering depression and separation anxiety when they're away from them. They're also razor-sharp, and will become bored and destructive if they are not entertained.

The best toys and enrichment activities for mini pigs provide both exercise and mental stimulation while mimicking their natural behaviors, such as rooting, foraging, burrowing, and exploring. They also need to be very strong. There are many great enrichment toys that you can create using repurposed items from your own home that would otherwise end up in the landfill.

The following are some DIY toys:

- **Almighty watering hole:** A kiddie pool filled with water can provide endless amounts of entertainment for your pig, who will splash around while also cooling down and getting hydrated. Put veggies into the pool for a "bobbing salad."

- **Mud wallow:** Dig a small trench in your yard and flood with water to make a shallow mud pit. Pigs love wallowing, rooting, and rolling in the mud. The mud also provides natural protection from the sun and insects.

- **String game:** String large pieces of fruits or vegetables from a rope suspended from a ceiling or outside porch. You can use a water bottle filled with a few treats so they have to flip it over with their nose to release them.

- **Rooting box:** Use a wooden crate or repurpose a sturdy plastic crate with river rocks and allow your pig to root through it to find treats. Great for both indoor and outdoor play.

- **Sandy treasure hunt:** Build a sandbox with old wood and fill it with soft sand. Hide treats such as air-popped popcorn in the sand.

- **Haystack:** Fill a cardboard box or large wooden crate with grass-based hay and hide treats in it. Your pig will love digging and searching through the grass to find them.

- **Treat jugs:** Turn an old plastic water jug or juice container into a pig toy by drilling holes in the sides and filling it with treats, such as oats or cheerios. Let your pig roll around to manipulate it to free the treats.

- **Paper games:** Let your pig shake and shred old newspapers, magazines, and phone books.

- **Recycle kid's toys:** Repurpose old children's toys and stuffed animals for pig enrichment toys.
- **Shredder:** Layer empty cardboard boxes for items such as crackers and cereal and hide treats in it. Let your pig shred the boxes to find the treats.

Grass-based hays can serve a multitude of purposes for your pet pig:

- Warm and insulating bedding for outdoor pens.
- Entertaining to play in and throw around.
- Great for chomping and eating.

Look for quality organic Timothy, orchard, oat, or grass-based hays. Pigs love alfalfa hay, but only provide in moderation because it contains more calories, which can pack on the pounds. Always store hay in a dry area where it can be aerated so it doesn't become moist or moldy.

To make the most environmentally conscious purchase, become friends with a local farmer in your area. Buying locally has a variety of benefits:

- Farm direct hay isn't packaged in plastic, as it is in the pet store.
- You can bring your own tub or container to fill.
- You are supporting a local farmer, which will in turn support your local community.
- It isn't shipped great distances to reach the pet store.
- Buying in large quantities is easier on the pocketbook.

7. Specialized Vet Care

Finding someone to treat your mini pig can be difficult. Some veterinarians won't treat mini pigs because they consider them to be livestock. City-dwellers may need to visit a large-animal specialist that treats farm animals.

To find a vet in your area:

- Ask a local animal clinic for a referral.
- Ask for a recommendation from a sanctuary, rescue, or breeder.
- Ask other pig owners who they use.
- Go online: The North American Potbellied Pig Association has a list of vets that treat pigs in the US and internationally (petpigs.com).

Because of their size and inability to climb, you will need a vehicle with significant cargo space to transport your pets to the vet, and a ramp to get them in and out. Pigs must be transported in a crate or enclosed space, and never in the back of a pickup truck, where they can jump out if spooked.

The following are some tips to keep your pig healthy:

- **Know the signs:** Prey animals by nature, mini pigs are very stoic and will try to hide sicknesses or illnesses. A telltale sign your pigs need to see the vet is a lack of appetite. It's rare that pigs won't eat. A change in behavior and activity level is often a signal they are in pain.
- **Annual checkups:** Preventative medicine is the greenest medicine! An annual examination will detect any potential problems and is also the time to bring up any dietary or exercise concerns and questions.
- **Hoof trimming:** Mini pig hooves grow similarly to human or dog fingernails and need to be trimmed regularly. While this can be performed by a vet, you can do it at home using a hard wire cutter, hoof trimming shears, or a Dremel rotary grinding tool.
- **Deworming:** Mini pigs are prone to having worms, and must be dewormed twice annually. This can be done either by a shot or medication given orally. You can purchase the dewormer and administer at home. Discuss dosage and treatment with your vet.

7.1 Spaying/neutering

Altering your piglet is the greenest care choice because it will prevent future health and behavioral problems. Intact sows are prone to mammary and uterine tumors and cancers in the reproductive tract, and spaying will greatly decrease the likelihood of those developing. An un-spayed female will mark her territory when she's in heat, which happens every three weeks.

Neutering a male is less about health than behavior: An intact boar will start exhibiting problem behaviors and sometimes become aggressive. To put it mildly, he will hump just about everything in sight, including other animals and furniture. He will also emit a musky smell.

By getting your pigs altered you are also reducing the pet overpopulation and decreasing the likelihood they will end up in a shelter or sanctuary — many people dump their unaltered pet piggies once they start exhibiting these undesirable behaviors.

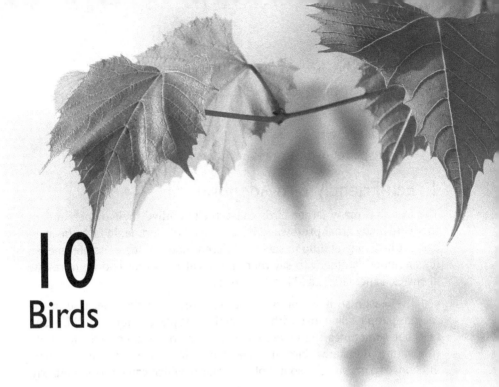

10
Birds

Long live birds! Birds are sensitive, inquisitive, and playful, which is why they're sometimes compared to toddlers who never grow up. These social creatures crave and love social time, so they need daily play and human socialization. Consider adopting two: Most birds in the wild are never alone and they love companionship, and many species thrive if they're paired with an avian buddy.

Birds by the numbers:

- In the US, 14.3 million pet birds are owned.
- The average companion bird will live in seven households over its lifetime.
- The average weight of a budgie is 30 to 35 grams.
- The percentage of body weight finches consume daily is 30 percent.
- One-third of the world's parrot species are threatened with extinction because of collecting for the pet trade and habitat loss.

Life spans for birds increase with body size. Here are the average life spans for common pet birds:

- Finch: 5 years

- Parakeet/budgie: 7 to 10 years
- Canary: 10 to 15 years
- Conure: 15 to 30 years
- Cockatiel: 15 to 20 years
- Large parrot (e.g., African Grey, Macaws): Up to 70 years

1. Eco-Friendly Bird Adoption

The fact that many larger birds can actually outlive their owners means there are many great pre-owned birds in need of a home. In fact, the average pet bird may end up in several different households in its lifetime, so it's an understatement to say there are great ones that end up in rescue agencies, sanctuaries, and local shelters.

The reason so many birds are surrendered is partially because of the reasons people fall in love with them in the first place. They sing, chirp, and talk, but sometimes the owner's expectations don't align with the bird's true nature. A talkative bird may speak in an incredibly high-pitched tone, or choose to imitate the sound of a car alarm, which can get tiring quickly.

Beyond their natural vocalizations, birds are very messy. They poop up to 30 times a day and fling food and seeds with zeal. They're talkative, curious, and destructive — like toddlers — which is why some owners get turned off.

As with other types of pets, adoption is the most environmentally conscious choice. That's because not only are you freeing up space for another homeless bird to take its place in the rescue, you're also sending a message that you don't support "bird mills," commercial breeding operations where thousands of birds are kept in filthy cages with little regard to their health and care. Those birds are often shipped thousands of miles to reach pet stores, which adds to the carbon footprint before they ever land in a family home.

To find a rescue bird for adoption, contact your local animal shelter or rescue group. An avian veterinarian or animal hospital may also have leads.

You can seek a small-scale local breeder in your area. A responsible breeder will —

- allow the parents to be part of the raising process;
- have a money-back guarantee and will take the bird back if it becomes ill;
- be able to provide references;
- be able to show the parents/breeding stock;

- have clean cages and provide high standards of health and hygiene for their birds; and
- screen adopters, to ensure their bird is going to a suitable home.

2. Home Hazards and Environmental Toxins

Birds have a delicate and complex respiratory system that makes them much more sensitive to toxins in the environment — and your home. Chronic exposure to toxins can irritate avian respiratory systems, or worse, cause their lungs to fatally hemorrhage.

The following sections discuss the most common household chemicals toxic to birds, and eco-friendly alternatives.

2.1 Teflon and nonstick cookware

Nonstick cookware made from the synthetic polymer polytetrafluoroethylene (PTFE) can be toxic to birds. These are often sold under the brand names Teflon and Silverstone. When the products are heated above 446 Fahrenheit (230 Celsius) they release fumes that are toxic and lethal to birds and can kill them within minutes. Almost all cookware products labeled "nonstick" contain PTFE, and should not be used around birds.

Eco-friendly alternatives: Use cast iron, ceramic, copper, and stainless steel pots and pans in the kitchen. Ensure these aren't treated with a nonstick surface.

Hidden Sources of Teflon

The chemical PTFE is present in dozens of common household appliances, and can be added as a coating on wires or other items. Ask the manufacturer if you're unclear if it's present in something you're buying.

The only guaranteed way to keep your birds safe is to avoid using PTFE items in your home altogether. The following are some common home items that contain the potentially lethal PTFE:

- Nonstick cookie sheets, muffin tins, pizza pans
- Self-cleaning ovens: Never use it with the bird in your home
- Drip pans
- Indoor cooktops and griddles
- Hair dryers

- Space heaters
- Deep fryers
- Waffle irons and panini presses
- Irons and ironing board covers
- Bread makers
- Popcorn makers

Make sure your bird's cage is always in a well-ventilated area with cross-ventilation — and never keep your bird in the kitchen.

2.2 Aerosol sprays and air fresheners

The particulate matter in aerosol sprays and air fresheners can cause breathing problems. This category includes hair sprays, dry shampoos, insecticides, and bug sprays. Scented sprays that make our homes smell nice (e.g., Febreze, air fresheners, perfumes) can seriously harm birds. Candles, potpourris, and plug-in fresheners that emit fumes are also irritants. Try to avoid using these items in your home altogether. If you do use them, make sure it's in a well-ventilated area, far away from your bird's cage.

2.3 Ammonia and bleach

The vapors in common home cleaners that use ammonia and bleach can cause irritation and lung inflammation. These are frequently found in kitchen and bathroom cleaners as well as glass, floor, oven, and brass cleaners.

Eco-friendly alternative: Only use nontoxic home cleaners, or make your own green formulations. See the download kit for eco-friendly cleaning recipes.

2.4 Smoke

Secondhand smoke from tobacco and marijuana as well as kitchen cooking smoke, can cause eye irritation and respiratory distress. Smoke from woodstoves and fireplaces can be harmful if the wood is treated with any chemicals.

Eco-friendly alternative: Keep your bird's cage away from any smoke sources.

2.5 Paint fumes

Fumes from house paints can cause respiratory distress. Birds can become sick if they chew on baseboards or toys that contain lead paint, which happens often in older homes.

Eco-friendly alternative: Only use paints that are low in volatile organic compounds (VOCs). Remove the bird from your home for a day or two if you're painting.

3. A Green Diet

While a lot of pet birds solely eat commercial pellets and seed mixes, they absolutely love and thrive on variety and fresh foods in their diet. That's because of where they originated: Birds in the wild spend their days foraging, cracking open seeds, and nibbling on fresh fruits.

If you're buying commercial seed mixes, buy organic when you can, but supplement their diet with these bird-friendly human foods:

- **Vegetables:** Carrots and their tops, corn, peas, broccoli, pumpkin, sweet potatoes, and bell peppers.
- **Greens:** Romaine lettuce, spinach, chard, and dandelion greens (these can be sourced from your home garden if not sprayed with pesticides).
- **Fruits:** Apples and pears (seeds removed), grapes, bananas, melons, mango, berries, and cantaloupes. Supply fruits only in moderation because of their high-sugar content.
- **Treats:** Unsalted nuts, cooked beans, scrambled eggs, and organic cereals (e.g., puffed grain and puffed wheat).

Avoid: Salt, caffeine, chocolate, avocados (pit and skin), cherries, pears, and peaches.

Even though some most birds are much smaller than other companion pets, there are still ways to minimize their environmental impact at feeding time.

That starts with dishing out less food. Many owners completely fill up the feeding dish with seeds, but that's much more than a pet bird needs nutritionally. A lot of food ends up being thrown out when birds only eat the top layer of their food and the rest is discarded.

Instead, portion food more appropriately by using a shallower dish and smaller portions. You can also make use of leftover seeds in your bird's dish by sharing the wealth, and using it to fill outdoor planters for wild birds.

The following are tips for "green" feeding:

- **Buy organic:** Whenever possible, source organic birdseed mixes and millet as well as vegetables grown without pesticides or insecticides.
- **Wash well:** Rinse produce thoroughly to remove pesticide residue.

- **Shop seasonally:** Avoid buying products that must be shipped long distances to market (e.g., squashes in fall, berries in summer, and sweet potatoes in winter).
- **Shop locally:** Visit farmers' markets for the freshest carrot tops and greens.
- **Compost:** Throw leftover seeds, millet, and produce into the compost or green bin to divert it from the landfill.

4. Cage Care

In terms of eco-friendliness, stainless steel is a solid choice for a cage as well as powder-coated cages. It's a one-time investment versus buying something made of plastic that can break and must be replaced in a short time. Wooden cages can become chew toys for curious birds, and aren't recommended for finches.

Sticks and branches of untreated wood in various thicknesses and diameter make great perches. Harder woods such as manzanita will last longer than softer woods. You can gather natural branches from outside to use in the cage as long as they aren't treated with pesticides or chemicals, and they're washed thoroughly beforehand. Plastic perches will be destroyed quickly.

Untreated plant pots made from unglazed ceramic and terra-cotta make great eco-friendly perches that will also help wear down your bird's nails naturally.

Birds thrive on social interaction so place your cage in an area of the home where they can interact with your family. The area should be well-ventilated, but also protected from extreme heat and cold fluctuations such as sunny or drafty windows.

Birds are notoriously messy and love to throw around the food in their cage — and a lot will inevitably end up on the floor. Birds can poop dozens of times a day so cage liners are critical. You'll be changing them often so using an environmentally friendly product will reduce your bird's carbon footprint.

Try these eco-friendly substrates:

- Recycled newspapers and magazines
- Paper towels made from postconsumer material

4.1 Eco-friendly cage cleaning

Besides changing the cage liner daily, birdcages need a thorough weekly cleaning. Guardians need to ensure they're using only nontoxic and environmentally friendly cleaning products that won't harm their bird's respiratory system. You can use plant-based, nontoxic commercial cleaning products as long as they are diluted and the cage is rinsed thoroughly afterwards.

You can easily make your own cage cleaner. Try these bird-friendly cleaners:

- Mix one part vinegar to two parts hot water.
- Heavy-duty cleaning paste: Mix 1/4 cup baking soda to 1 quart water.
- General cleaner: Mix 1/3 cup baking soda to a gallon of water.
- Grapefruit cleaner: 20 drops of grapefruit seed extract mixed into 32-ounce spray bottle of water.
- Steam cleaners used only with plain water.
- Mild nontoxic dishwashing liquid mixed with hot water, rinsed well.

5. Exercise and Enrichment

In nature, birds can fly hundreds of miles each day, and spend their waking hours foraging, digging, and playing. Companion birds in the home obviously don't log those kind of flight hours so it's imperative to provide them with room to spread their wings and enrichment toys to satisfy those natural instincts.

Just like humans, birds can get overweight and even obese, a phenomenon referred to as "Perch Potatoes." Overweight avians can suffer from heart disease and plaque in the arteries and their life spans can be drastically reduced if they don't get enough exercise.

The best life for a bird is one that's spent with lots of time outside of its cage. This section provides eco-friendly strategies to keep your birds lean and green!

5.1 Safe-flight space

The best way to exercise and entertain your birds is giving them a safe flight space. It's also the most environmentally conscious method of enrichment: It requires no products or money.

Creating an indoor or outdoor aviary or flight-safe room requires bird-proofing an area to ensure they don't harm themselves or damage your home. Rooms such as hallways, living rooms, and screened porches make more suitable aviaries than bathrooms and kitchens, where water and heating elements can pose hazards.

The following are some ways to bird-proof a room:

- Turn off ceiling fan.
- Remove or cover mirrors.

- Close windows.
- Pull down shades or blinds.
- Close fireplace.
- Cover electrical cords to discourage chewing.
- Remove any fragile objects (e.g., picture frames or vases).
- Remove other pets from the room.
- Close doors to the room to prevent escape.

5.2 Easy and eco-friendly enrichment

The best enrichment toys are ones that allow your bird to act on its natural behaviors, including foraging, chewing, preening, climbing, hopping, and shredding.

There are dozens of items you can provide that don't have a large environmental footprint, including many you likely already have in your home and yard. Switch them out often to decrease boredom:

- **Splash time:** Use an unglazed terra-cotta or ceramic dish to create a shallow birdbath to splash around in.
- **Cool down fun:** Put a large ice cube on a side plate and let them rattle it around.
- **Tear apart:** Reuse pages of newspaper, old phone books, paper towel rolls, cardboard egg cartons, and small cardboard boxes as shredding toys.
- **Bring in the outside:** Well-washed and chemical-free fruit tree branches make great perches in different sizes and shapes. These help birds to exercise their feet and legs.
- **Wood chews:** Put pieces of untreated wood inside their cage. Drill holes into a piece and stuff it with several treats. Pinecones also make good chews.
- **Natural fun:** String natural fiber rope from the top of or across the cage for climbing.
- **Treat bundles:** Wrap snacks inside a brown paper bag or paper towel made from recycled paper and hang from the top or side of the cage.
- **Suspended fun:** Hang a natural rice cake from an unpainted wooden spoon from the top of the cage.

At the pet store, look for toys made from natural materials that are nontoxic and come from sustainable sources (e.g., straw, untreated wood, wicker). Toys from natural materials can often be recycled, composted, or put into your lawn trimmings container so they won't end up in the landfill.

6. Bird-friendly vets

Birds are stoic, and by the time they display signs of illness it can mean they are very sick, or close to death. That's why it's critical to seek an avian specialist to care for your bird. These are veterinarians in clinical practice who have undergone additional training to specialize in avian care. Expect these practitioners to be more expensive than a vet that treats cats and dogs.

Finding an avian specialist in your area may be difficult so ask around. Local bird rescues and shelters will be able to provide a vet care reference, and veterinary hospitals often have an avian specialist.

The Association of Avian Veterinarians has an online directory that lists board-certified vets in your area (aav.org).

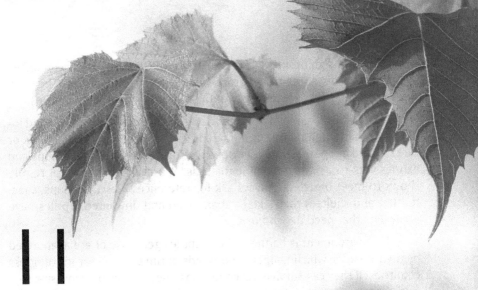

11
Reptiles and Amphibians

With origins including African deserts and South American rainforests, the carbon footprint required to keep some popular reptile and amphibian species are much larger than the average dog or cat. They need specialized lighting and heating to thrive — and trying to replicate a reptile's natural environment can be exponentially more complicated and costly than caring for other pets. This chapter explores ways to reduce the carbon footprint of your turtle or tortoise, lizard, iguana, snake, tree frog, and bearded dragon.

1. Eco-Friendly Adoption

While the thought of wild-caught exotics brings to mind idyllic images of Indiana Jones-type explorers foraging the wilderness, that's not the case. Thousands of exotics are sourced for pet stores each year through the wildlife trade, which causes a great deal of disruption and harm to natural ecosystems and native populations when the creatures are removed from their habitat.

Of equal environmental harm are exotic pet mills, where reptiles and amphibians are produced in large numbers for profit, often in substandard conditions with little concern for their welfare. Both wild-caught and milled

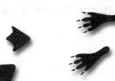

animals have a significantly larger carbon footprint because they are often shipped great distances to pet stores, domestically or overseas. The creatures are often packed into small containers and many will die in transit.

The greenest source of reptiles are those that are captive-born and locally bred, although neither is a guarantee of environmental standards or care. To find a reputable breeder, speak to local herp clubs and groups and exotics vets to ask for recommendations. You can also visit local reptile shows to meet breeders. Always ask for references. Rescue groups, sanctuaries, and shelters that take in abandoned and unwanted reptiles have great pets that need new homes.

The environment is harmed when reptiles get loose or are abandoned by their owners, which happens thousands of times each year in countless countries. If they can survive the conditions, they can become invasive species, damage the ecosystem, and threaten the natural order.

A number of North American municipalities have strict bylaws in place regarding wild and captive reptile species alike. Some prohibit the ownership of captive reptiles, including snakes and small sea turtles, outright. The American Veterinary Medical Association and Center for Disease Control each oppose keeping certain reptiles as pets. Learn about your local area's legalities before purchasing any reptile.

2. Veterinary Care

The most common medical issues for reptiles are related to inadequate husbandry, nutrition, and housing — and these rarely happen in isolation. Reliant on thermoregulation, their physiologies and metabolism stop functioning efficiently without proper heat and light. For example, diurnal reptiles that are active during the day require ultraviolet-B (UVB) light exposure to make the vitamin D3 needed to absorb calcium. A UVB light deficiency can quickly lead to a calcium deficiency, which causes serious health problems, such as bone disease.

The closer you can replicate their ideal temperature, lighting, and humidity requirements the longer and happier their lives will be.

2.1 Seek a specialist

Whether it's a gecko, snake, or tree frog, the physiology of reptiles and amphibians are radically different from a cat or dog. That's the reason why many vets won't accept reptile patients: It's out of their comfort zone and they've had virtually no training or education about these pets.

"The majority of veterinarians are inept at treating reptiles," says Dr. Anthony Pilny, a veterinarian with the Center for Avian and Exotic Medicine in New York City.

It's essential to seek an exotics specialist or someone who has undergone training and certification. Another reason to find someone experienced? Herps are hard to diagnose. These are prey creatures who will go to great lengths to hide their illness, as not to appear vulnerable to potential predators. From an environmental standpoint, specialist care is also the greenest: Someone who understands the nutritional and care requirements of reptiles will ensure they are in optimal health and be able to identify potential health issues before they become serious and require treatment.

How to find a reptile specialist:

- Local herp society, pet clubs, and hobbyists.
- Vet clinics. Check to see if the vet is involved in any herp associations or professional organizations.
- Rescues and animal shelters.
- Pet stores and local breeders.
- Online reviews.
- The Association of Reptilian and Amphibian Veterinarians (ARAV) has an online directory of North American and international members (arav.org/find-a-vet).

2.2 Zoonotic concerns

Zoonotic pathogens and parasites are common in many reptiles and can be transmitted to pet owners through handling. The most common offender is salmonella, but the risks are decreased if you keep your reptile healthy, says exotics specialist Dr. Adrian Walton, from Dewdney Animal Hospital.

"The type of salmonella reptiles carry can make people very sick and reptiles are more likely to shed the bacteria when sick or neglected," Dr. Walton says.

Proper handling, hygiene, and common sense greatly decrease contamination risks, including washing your hands after handling your reptiles, their cage, and their food. Keep their enclosure clean and don't let them walk on your kitchen counters or anywhere food is prepared or consumed.

3. Enclosures

Environmentally conscious reptile keeping begins with what you use for housing. Instead of using a plastic or resin cage, choose a material such as solid glass that will last a lifetime and won't rot or fall apart.

Instead of buying new, consider repurposing a tank that was used for another type of pet. A cracked fish aquarium can find new life as a terrarium for a non-amphibious reptile. Also consider buying a gently used secondhand cage. Online buy-and-sell marketplaces such as Craigslist, eBay, and Kijiji are full of listings for pre-owned enclosures that are nearly new. You can also sell yours when you're done with it — upcycling it again.

The ideal enclosure should include natural items that enhance your reptile's mental and physical enrichment and mimic the behaviors it would exhibit in the wild, such as burrowing, foraging, digging, climbing, balancing, and stretching.

"Make sure you are providing as much space as you can and breaking up the line of sight with rocks and branches to encourage them to move around," says Carrie Kish, Director of Reptelligence.

3.1 All-natural vivariums

While there are many artificial plants, grasses, and other greenery available to mimic a natural setting for your reptile, you can opt for the real deal by creating an all-natural vivarium.

These terrariums are constructed using layers of natural substrates, plants, moss, and organic matter. They function as a self-contained and aesthetically pleasing ecosystem in your home. The key to these types of natural enclosures is starting with an appropriate substrate and drainage; otherwise, it runs the risk of creating mold.

It is labor-intensive to create a vivarium, but believers say there is much less maintenance required for the "bio active" set up, and it smells better. There is less waste because the substrate will not need to be replaced. Instead, you will need to add more soil as the existing matter decomposes and composts.

Short of going 100 percent natural, you can still put your green thumb to work by planting live greenery inside your enclosure. Live plants are a literal green step to mimic the natural environment while also providing enrichment. Turtles love swimming through aquatic plants, which also add oxygen into the water. Chameleons enjoy climbing and exploring a Ficus tree. Not all plants are equally green: Some require extra energy-sucking broad-spectrum lighting to thrive.

The type of plants that are appropriate depends on two important factors: The species you keep and the environment you keep them in. Not all plants are reptile-safe, so seek the advice of your vet or your local herp club before introducing anything new. Live plants may not be suitable for reptiles that chow down on whatever organic matter you put into their cages.

Think about the individual type of enclosure and the conditions inside it. Temperature, light, heat, moisture, and humidity are all key considerations. The requirements of a desert plant are vastly different than an orchid, air plant, or ivy.

Planting within your terrarium begins with adding a layer of soil free of phosphates and fertilizer, and choosing items that are reptile safe. Be careful where you source your plants: Make sure they are organic and in-secticide- and pesticide-free. Consider growing the plant outside of the enclosure for up to six weeks before adding it to reduce the risk of any pesticide residue.

Short of creating a whole vivarium, you can add items from the natural world into your terrarium to create a habitat that will more closely resemble their home habitat and provide enrichment:

- Pesticide-free branches pruned from fruit trees can be used for decoration, and bound together to create climbing apparatuses. Ensure the tree wasn't sprayed with chemicals.
- Driftwood that has been sunbaked for many years adds visual interest to an enclosure and can be used for climbing.
- Natural river rocks work well for decoration and basking.

Anything put into the terrarium must first be washed in warm water. Avoid household cleaners, which contain chemicals that can hurt your pet's health and water sources. Before adding wood, you can bake it at 200 to 250 degrees Fahrenheit (95 to 120 degrees Celsius) for half an hour to kill any bacteria, bugs, and mites. Avoid sapwoods, which will smoke in the oven.

3.2 Substrates and eco-friendly bedding

This is one category where it's quite easy to go green. Most common cage substrates, cage liners, and bedding originate from nature or are by-products of manufacturing a natural product. Many can be diverted from the landfill by composting or recycling.

Consider these eco-friendly beddings:

- **Natural soils:** Sand, potting soil, bark, or mulch can be composted with your garden waste. If your reptile is a carnivore, do not use this compost on food plants, only flowers and ornamental gardens.
- **Bark:** Sometimes from fir trees, this can be used for upwards of a year, provided it's cleaned every few months by soaking it in hot water and fully drying. It's also compostable.
- **Aspen:** Made from a renewable resource, snakes and lizards love burrowing and bedding in these all-natural shavings.
- **Carpets and felt mats:** While not inherently eco-friendly, these long-lasting products can be cut to fit any sized terrarium and can be cleaned and reused many times. Many are washing machine safe.

- **Coconut fiber:** A natural by-product of coconut processing, this absorbent bedding made from husks and fiber can be composted. Good for burrowing reptiles.

- **Sphagnum moss:** Can be rinsed and reused up to four times. It's compostable or can be put into yard trimmings.

- **Newspaper:** Though not the most aesthetically pleasing, you can reuse old newspaper to line enclosures, and recycle it afterwards.

3.3 Go green when you clean

A thorough weekly cleaning is necessary for the cage, decorations, and substrates and will help your reptile live a healthier life with less risk of skin and bacterial infections.

Exercise caution when choosing cage cleaners. Reptiles can suffer respiratory sensitivities and distress from household cleaning products that contain harsh chemicals so it's extra important that these products aren't used in their terrariums. This is especially true of frogs, which can absorb chemicals through their permeable skin.

Vinegar and hot water works well for general cage cleaning. You can use hot water with a drop of nontoxic dish soap to detach stubborn organic debris. If left on for upwards of 20 minutes, hydrogen peroxide makes a green alternative to chlorine and other disinfectants.

If you are purchasing a commercial cleaner, look for formulations that are —

- biodegradable,
- 100 percent natural,
- fragrance-free, and
- free of Volatile Organic Compounds (VOCs) and chlorine.

To reduce the risk of bacteria (e.g., salmonella) spreading to humans, always clean enclosures and bedding away from any areas where food is prepared and wash your hands afterwards.

4. Heating and Lighting for Enclosures

Environmentally conscious reptile keeping begins with the species you choose. Species from North America typically thrive in a much more temperate climate than desert or South American species, and will not need as much electricity-gobbling heating to thrive.

Some lower-impact species include herbivorous pets such as corn snakes, frogs, salamanders, and box turtles. Nocturnal species, including some geckos, will have less intensive lighting requirements, although they still may need a source of ultraviolet light. Size is another consideration. Even if a tiny species requires heating, it will be in a smaller enclosure that takes less electricity to heat.

Reptiles are ectothermic, meaning they absorb heat from external sources to regulate and maintain their body temperature. In nature, many reptiles will bask on sunny rocks during the day for warmth. In your home, you will use heating and lighting in conjunction to achieve a target temperature range.

The biggest environmental impact of this group of pets is the energy used for heating and lighting in their enclosures, but the importance of these two items can't be understated. Without them, reptiles can suffer a range of negative health effects, vitamin deficiencies, and even early deaths.

4.1 Timers and thermostats

One of the largest energy savers is the use of timers. When attached to thermostats, timers hooked up to heat sources will allow you to keep the enclosure at the perfect temperature zone around the clock without wasting electricity. It also allows you to drop the temperature appropriately at night, to replicate how an ecosystem is cooler after the sun goes down.

Timers can also be used to control lighting. Energy is frequently wasted when owners forget to turn off lights in the evening. A timer will do this automatically and save energy in the process.

4.2 Lighting

Terrarium lighting should mimic conditions in the wild where there is approximately 12 hours each day of sunlight and darkness.

Jesse De Luca, National Reptile Specialist for Rolf C. Hagen Inc., recommends having lights on for 10 to 14 hours a day. "Beyond that you're wasting energy and then also that bulb is going to burn out faster," he says.

You can be more energy efficient in your lighting by doing the following:

- Put all lights on timers.
- Buy the appropriate lighting for your species (e.g., desert bulbs for desert species).
- Use the correct wattage.
- Source high-quality lighting because it will last longer.

If you are not using the lighting for heat, or the climate where you live is naturally warm enough, you can use LED lights, which have a long life span, are easy on energy, and don't give off any extra heat.

Reptiles, especially those from sunny desert climates, require ultraviolet-B (UVB) light to synthesize vitamin D3. Without it they can suffer severe calcium deficiencies, bone issues, and metabolic diseases.

"Proper full spectrum lighting is very important in the complete care of many reptiles. When you keep them indoors without the correct UVB light — this often leads to significant problems," says Animal House of Chicago's Dr. Byron J.S. De la Navarre, past President of the Association of Reptilian and Amphibian Veterinarians.

Sunlight coming through your home's windows doesn't provide enough UVB because the majority of the rays are filtered through the windowpanes and the enclosure. To protect and promote your reptile's health, source a special UVB light for its enclosure. This full-spectrum lighting must be replaced twice annually because the bulbs will stop producing the UV after six to eight months.

These lights come in several formats, including compact fluorescent, linear fluorescent, mercury vapor, and combination lights that emit UV light and a heat source. Compact fluorescents (CFLs) are the most efficient — they use less energy, have lower watts, and last longer than conventional bulbs.

Access to real, unfiltered sunshine is a health-boosting measure for reptiles that has a zero-carbon footprint. Exposure to the sun, even if it's only for ten minutes at a time, will allow them to store up vitamin D.

"The sun is free, always available, and is absolutely life-sustaining for reptiles," says Dr. Anthony Pilny.

The key to doing this is safety: If you're taking your reptiles outside, they must be supervised so they can't hurt themselves, wander away, or become prey.

Outdoor time can come in the form of a simple wander around the yard, or a deck or screened porch, provided it's secure. You can also repurpose a children's wading pool or sandbox to contain your reptile outside. Reptile enthusiasts in warmer climates can build outdoor exercise areas and enclosures for their pet to soak up the sun year-round.

4.3 Heating

Some reptile species require an additional heat source to keep them in the correct temperature zone, which can be provided by a combination of heat-bulbs, ceramic heat sources, and under-tank heaters. All sources should be hooked up to a thermostat to avoid wasting energy.

Heat and basking lights are high-watt heat bulbs, which emit both light and heat, mimic the sun, and are placed over the basking spot in the habitat. These lightweight bulbs are less efficient than ceramic sources because they burn out easily. To save energy, only use the wattage required for your reptile, and use a timer so it can turn off automatically in the evening. Under-tank, ceramic, or night-heat lamps can be used if heat is needed overnight.

Placing a heat-absorbent material under your basking area, such as stone, will retain more heat in the enclosure and allow for a lower wattage on your heat lamp. Make sure to monitor the temperature to ensure the surface doesn't get too hot.

Under-tank heat sources are much more efficient than heat lamps so choose these whenever possible versus incandescent bulbs to save on energy. These can be connected to a thermostat or herpstat to keep the tank warmer or cooler at night, depending on your reptile's needs.

Ceramic heat lamps are radiant bulbs that are much more energy-efficient than heat lamps because they produce heat with no light. They last much longer because they are much more heavy-duty than a delicate glass bulb and don't have a filament that can burn out. You can use this heat source in combination with energy-efficient lighting (e.g., LEDs) to reduce your electricity consumption.

5. Feeding

If the reptile kingdom were a group of friends, they would have a hard time picking a restaurant to eat dinner. That's because their diets are vastly different: Some are strict carnivores, while others are insectivores, herbivores, and vegetarians.

The "greenest" choice you can make is by choosing a species that doesn't eat meat so you can eliminate the carbon footprint associated with producing and shipping that protein. (Not to mention the "ick" factor of feeding frozen, dead animals to your carnivores.) One way to reduce the environmental impact of these meat-loving herps is to raise your own mice or rats for feeding, but again, this is not for the faint-hearted.

Here's how to make the greenest choices for every type of reptile and amphibian:

- **Know your herp:** How much food does it need? Does it eat every day? Are there foods it doesn't like? By being in tune with your herp's schedule and understanding its preferences, you can reduce food waste, especially for species that don't eat every day.
- **Keep it seasonal:** The amount of food your reptile needs can change depending on what time of year it is and its activity level during

those months. Seasonal also applies to shopping for food (e.g., source local squashes in fall and leafy lettuces in summer).

- **Keep it local:** For herbivores, buy local fruits and vegetables whenever possible, and organic. Ask at your grocery store or farmers' market for discarded green tops and beet greens for your herbivores.

- **Grow your own:** Eliminate the transportation footprint associated with food production by producing your own meals. For herbivores that could mean growing leafy greens and lettuces, or growing grasses.

- **Create a colony:** For the same reason herp owners keep gardens for reptile food, many people are cutting out the trips to the pet store and raising their own insect colonies. Whether it's crickets, roaches, or wingless fruit flies, this completely removes the carbon footprint associated with packaging food and delivering it to pet stores.

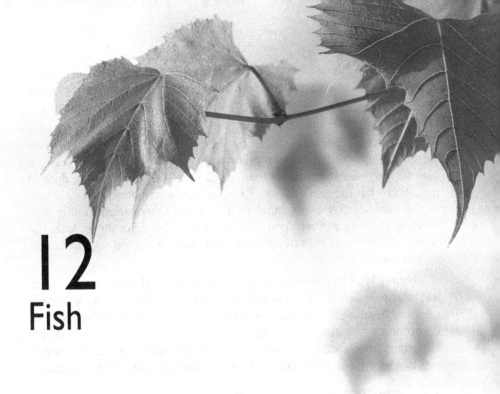

12
Fish

An estimated 13.6 million US households own a combined 105-million freshwater and saltwater fish, according to the American Pet Products Association.[1] The popularity of home aquarium keeping has surged in recent years, thanks partly to the Disney film *Finding Nemo*, which follows a clownfish trying to reunite with his son after his capture from the Great Barrier Reef. What the animated film didn't illustrate is that hobby aquarium keeping is far from child's play. Many species require specialized care and energy-consuming lighting, heating, circulation, and filter systems.

1. Choosing Your Fish

Fish sold in the marine aquarium industry have many hidden environmental costs. The species you choose, how it is harvested, and where it comes from all factor into the overall eco-impact.

1.1 Wild versus farmed

Millions of tropical aquarium fish are wild-caught each year, according to the United Nations Environment Programme's World Conservation Monitoring

---

1 "Pet Industry Market Size & Ownership Statistics," American Pet Products Association (APPA), accessed January 2016. americanpetproducts.org/press_industrytrends.asp

Centre. It's a major issue because harvesting directly from fragile marine ecosystems can take a staggering environmental toll. This is especially true for the removal of saltwater ornamentals, where native fish populations and coral reefs are inevitably harmed during collection.

A damning report on wild fish harvesting by the UN found that fishermen in countries such as Indonesia routinely squirt cyanide into reefs to stun fish to make it easier for them to capture. The nearly lethal dose of poison can kill the reef and cause declines in other native species. Many of the fish die after being purchased in North America, presuming they survived the long and cramped shipping process from Southeast Asia. The report said the survival rate could be less than one in ten for fish caught with cyanide.[2]

If there is a silver lining, it's that the obscenely high death rate of chemical catches is actually turning fishermen off the practice. More and more responsible wild-catch operations support conservation practices and local economies, impose catch limits, and use hand-nets. As a consumer, it's important to research the species you're interested in to find out how it was harvested, and seek only wild sources that are sustainably managed.

1.2 Saltwater versus freshwater

It is much harder to breed saltwater tropical species in a farm-cultured, captive environment, but there are some companies that are producing aquacultured saltwater fish to satiate the demand of environmentally conscientious aquarists.

Through its Florida marine hatchery, which is the biggest in North America, Oceans, Reefs & Aquariums (ORA) sells many species that are normally wild harvested. Its goal is to eventually have a 100 percent farmed reef aquarium, to conserve the natural reef habitats around the world.

Freshwater fish are a much more eco-friendly choice because 90 percent are farm raised. Many of the farms are in Florida so the carbon footprint for shipping in North America is much smaller compared to species shipped from overseas.

Another benefit is that many freshwater ornamentals can thrive in cooler waters so you don't need an aquarium setup that requires heaters. You can reduce your carbon footprint by sourcing species that do well in temperate tanks compared to their tropical counterparts.

1.3 Ethical and local sourcing

An even greener choice is sourcing fish bred locally. Ask your local pet store or fish hobby group for contacts for small-scale breeders in your

---

2 "From Ocean to Aquarium," Colette Wabnitz, Michelle Taylor, Edmund Green, and Tries Razak, United Nations Environment Programme (UNEP), accessed January 2016. unep.org/PDF/From_Ocean_To_Aquarium_report.pdf

area. James A. Krause, owner of the aquarium store Rivers to Reef, says fish that don't have to endure shipping from long distances are often healthier and less stressed.

"They are typically used to local water quality parameters which can increase success rates when taking them home," Krause says.

You need to do your homework to find out which wild-caught species come from sustainable sources, and unfortunately pet and aquarium stores don't always have the answer. The organization Reef Protection International has an online Reef Fish Guide to help consumers make environmentally sustainable fish choices (reefprotect.org/fish_guide_index.htm). It evaluates hundreds of marine species on criteria including the collection method, wild population, harm to natural ecosystems, and suitability for captive breeding.

2. Environmentally Responsible Coral

Heralded as the "rainforest of the sea," coral reefs are diverse and fragile ecosystems that support a staggering amount of marine life. In your home reef aquarium, coral and live rocks not only look beautiful, they purify the water and provide shelter.

Harvesting coral from the wild puts a significant strain on these precious ecosystems, 30 percent of which are already seriously threatened because of overfishing and destructive harvesting practices, according to Reef Protection International.[3] Up to 12 million stony corals are harvested, transported, and sold annually, according to the United Nations Environment Programme's World Conservation Monitoring Centre. Many countries have few, if any, regulations about ethical and sustainable harvesting.[4]

To minimize harm, seek coral that is farm-raised and generated through the process of "fragging," which uses a small piece of acclimated coral from a parent colony. These are often called "aquacultured corals." Aside from avoiding the carbon footprint of shipping from overseas, these are created sustainably and don't impact natural reefs.

These aquaculture corals or live rocks are grown in a captive environment for several generations. Some are grown in greenhouses or farms across the US, typically in warmer states, or on live racks in an ocean environment in countries such as Fiji and Indonesia.

The greenest way to source aquacultured corals is to look for organized "frag swaps" in your area where hobbyists and clubs buy, trade, and sell domestically cultured corals to other reef enthusiasts. Websites

---

3 "Coral Reefs at Risk: Collecting Gone Wild," Reef Protection International, accessed January 2016. reefprotect.org/reef_crisis.htm
4 "From Ocean to Aquarium," Colette Wabnitz, Michelle Taylor, Edmund Green, and Tries Razak, United Nations Environment Programme (UNEP), accessed January 2016. unep.org/PDF/From_Ocean_To_Aquarium_report.pdf

such as AsapAquarium.com have online listings of free swap events across North America.

3. Tanks

Whether you choose to keep a Tabletop Nano Aquarium or an elaborate planted reef, many factors play into how much energy your home setup uses. Consider the species, plants, and corals; and the heaters, chillers, filters, and lighting required to mimic the natural ecosystem.

3.1 Size

"Go big or go home" should not be your motto when setting up your home aquarium. Although it is crucial to the health and well-being of each species to follow the guidelines for proper water and space requirements, you don't need to go overboard when it comes to the size of the aquarium.

The larger the tank is, the more lighting, heating, and energy-drawing accessories it needs. By using only the space you need, and using equipment that is appropriately powered for that space, you will not waste energy.

3.2 Lighting

The biggest energy draw in a home aquarium is lighting (about 40 percent), but environmental savings can be had by selecting efficient systems and controlling the number of hours they are in use. Lighting requirements vary dramatically by what the tank contains:

- **Basic:** An aquarium without plants or corals will not require broad-spectrum light for photosynthesis, so lower wattage and fewer hours of lighting are acceptable.
- **Coral:** Full-spectrum, high-intensity lighting is needed to support the healthy growth of live rock or coral.
- **Plants:** The faster-growing and more delicate the plant, the more broad-spectrum lighting it requires to promote photosynthesis. Some varieties need 12 hours of light a day to thrive.

The biggest energy saver is switching from fluorescent lighting fixtures to light-emitting diodes (LEDs) whenever possible. LEDs deliver a more intense light output and use a fraction of the power — up to 70 percent less than fluorescents. Because they emit less heat than power compacts or halides, the need for a cooling fan is also eliminated.

They cost more upfront but LEDs last significantly longer than T5 or T8 fluorescents or incandescent lamps, which need to be replaced approximately every six to nine months. With 10 hours of daily usage, some Fluval LEDs can last upwards of 50,000 hours — that's 13 years. Higher-powered LED systems have the spectrum and intensity to support plant and coral growth, but not all are created equal. Ask the manufacturer what the specific bulb is capable of.

Fish respond better to having consistent periods of lighting. Putting your aquarium lighting on a timer guarantees your fish always get exactly the right amount of light without ever wasting energy. It will also prevent excess algae growth, which is sped up by excessive light. You can time your lighting hours to coincide with when you are actually home to enjoy the aquarium.

Reducing the daily hours of aquarium lighting is another way to shrink your eco-footprint. Most tropical fishes and plants will do well with 8 hours of light per day rather than 12.

3.3 Heaters and chillers

With many species originating from the warm waters of countries such as Indonesia and the Philippines, heating is a nonnegotiable component of tropical aquariums. Heaters and chillers typically account for 30 to 35 percent of a typical aquarium's energy consumption. There are three main ways to conserve energy:

- **Don't overheat:** Know what the requirements are for the species and don't heat more than that temperature.

- **Properly powered:** Have enough wattage to heat the volume of water by the proper amount of degrees compared to the room temperature. An underpowered heater in a large tank will be forced to run constantly, increasing energy consumption.

- **Tank placement:** Place your home aquarium in a heated and central location where it won't be subject to temperature swings and extremes such as sunny windows or drafty doors. Your heater will be forced to work overtime if your aquarium is in a part of your home that gets lots of cold air. Keeping a lid on your aquarium will prevent heat from escaping in cooler months.

3.4 Water filters and air pumps

The typical aquarium energy consumption for water filters and air pumps is about 15 percent. These components use less power than heating and lighting, but you can still reduce their carbon footprint by following simple guidelines:

- Choose energy-efficient equipment — compare models.

- Clean pumps and hoses regularly to keep them in good working order.

- Use appropriately sized devices in your tank.

Using equipment meant for a larger setup will waste power, and under-powered gear will have to work harder and will burn out faster, meaning it will need replaced more often.

3.5 Tank cleaning and water changes

Maintaining a healthy aquatic environment for your fish will decrease harmful toxins and extend their lives. Doing regular partial tank changes removes organic-waste pollutants and improves water clarity, which creates a healthier ecosystem. The obvious environmental impact of tank changes is the water consumption, but there are simple steps that will both improve water quality and the time in between water changes:

- **Filters:** A filter in good working order will decrease organic pollutants including gases, waste particles, odors, and debris that decrease water quality. Cleaning your filters and replacing them regularly will keep the water cleaner and prevent cloudiness.

- **Green aquarium cleaning:** Never use commercial window cleaners to clean an empty tank because they contain ammonia, which is toxic to fish. Soaps can also leave toxic residues. For glass aquarium cleaning, use a solution of hot water with vinegar. You can use newspaper to wipe and recycle it afterwards.

- **Home pollutants:** Airborne chemical particulate in home cleaners and cosmetics can contaminate aquarium water and poison your fish. Insect repellents, hairspray, perfumes, and aerosol air fresheners should never be used around fish tanks.

Instead of pouring tank water down the drain, give it new life by using it on your lawn or home garden. The waste produced by fish converts to nitrogen, which in turn will fertilize and enrich your plants (recommended for ornamental gardens, shrubs, and flowers, but not food plants). Don't use the water —

- if your tank was, or fish were, recently treated with chemicals or medications;

- if aquarium salt was used; and

- on indoor plants because the used water can emit an unpleasant smell in your home.

A growing number of hobbyists are experimenting with water recycling through home aquaponics, a sustainable food system that couples aquaculture with hydroponics. This ancient form of aquatic gardening dates back to the Aztec era.

In an aquaponic aquarium, the fish waste, uneaten food, and algae that normally degrade water quality are pumped out of the tank and used as liquid fertilizer for plants growing on top. The greenery absorbs those nitrates as nutrients. The cleaned and oxygenated water is returned down to the tank through the plants' roots, where the process starts all over again.

Because of its efficiency in recycling water and eliminating waste, vegetables grown in an aquaponic system require only a fraction of what's normally required for water. The organic growing system requires no chemicals or synthetic fertilizers.

Commercial aquaponics systems that raise fish (e.g., tilapia) for food can be the size of a football field but there are much smaller home and nano setups designed to grow organic fruits and vegetables using your home hobby aquarium. There are plenty of online resources on DIY aquaponics if you want to start your own.

4. Benefits of Live Plants

Adding natural plants to your aquatic environment is literally the greenest way to keep your fish healthy and happy and has a multitude of benefits:

- **Aeration:** Through photosynthesis, plants naturally absorb carbon dioxide and release oxygen into the atmosphere, which fish use in respiration. Adding plants can reduce the need for air pumps and air stones.
- **Behavior:** Live plants act as natural shelter, shade, and cover and will reduce aggression and stress in your stock. Timid species will appreciate the hiding spaces.
- **Absorbs waste:** Plants will naturally absorb and remove fish waste, including nutrients such as phosphates, nitrates, and ammonium. Actively growing plants will filter this biological waste, reducing the frequency of water changes.
- **Algae control:** Algae thrives on waste nutrients produced by fish, but live plants will absorb those micro-elements instead, starving out the algae. The result? Less algae and no need for harsh algaecides.
- **Eliminates garbage:** Silk and plastic artificial plants can look life-like, but will eventually end up in the landfill. Unwanted live plants can be composted or collected along with your yard trimmings.

Some plants require higher-spectrum lighting for up to 12 hours, which will add to the carbon footprint of your setup. Others will thrive in lower-light conditions and LED bulbs. Generally speaking, the faster growing and more delicate the plant, the more light it will require.

Your local aquarium store can provide guidance on which submersible plants are appropriate for your species and tank setup. Introduce hardier species in the beginning — these will eat the most algae — and then add in more sensitive plants.

4.1 Battling algae naturally

Algae is the thorn in every aquarist's side, and some home hobbyists have abandoned their pursuits over it when frustrations spill over. The growth of algae is accelerated by access to food and light so limiting those factors will result in less algae. Beyond adding live plants to your aquarium, there are other natural ways to inhibit stubborn algae growth:

- **Reducing light:** Place your aquarium away from natural light sources (e.g., sunny windows or skylights). Use timers to control the amount of tank lighting. Natural plants require a certain amount of broad-spectrum lighting, but timers ensure they are only lit for the period required. Placing floating plants on the surface of the tank can also cut off the light supply to algae.

- **Feed appropriately:** Algae multiplies when it has access to large quantities of fish waste and uneaten fish food, both of which are by-products of overfeeding. Cut off this supply chain by not overfeeding your fish, and removing uneaten food from the aquarium using a fine net. A recommended feeding guideline is to only provide as much as your species can eat within two minutes.

- **Adding competition:** Scrubbing pads are designed to go to war with tank algae, but you can also let something else do the work for you. There are various snails and bottom-dwelling herbivorous fish for freshwater tanks that will happily munch on your unwanted algae. In saltwater tanks you can introduce macroalgae species to battle algae. Not all algae-eaters will live in harmony in every aquarium so speak to an expert to see if it's a good fit.

A final word of warning: Algae can also be the result of other tank issues so it's worth investigating the cause before introducing any species to control the unwanted organic growth.

5. The Green Good-bye

The movie *Finding Nemo* escalated the popularity of home aquaculture but also had a darker, unintended side effect: Kids flushing fish down the toilet to "free them" back to the ocean. However, experts warn that flushing live fish, or releasing them back into public waterways in general, has disastrous consequences for the environment and fish welfare.

Most flushed fish die of shock from the chemicals in the septic system or, if it makes it that far, the sewage treatment plant. Fish "freed" into waterways can introduce potentially harmful pathogens and disease that can pollute the water and harm wild-fish populations.

If the fish survives, it can become an invasive species and take over native populations and decimate biodiversity. The Indo-Pacific lionfish, known for their insatiable appetite, are responsible for a 65 percent decline in native coral reef fish in the Bahamas over a two-year period.[5]

If you need to re-home fish, consider donating them to a local aquarium or pet store, or see if a pound or rescue will take them. Talk to a fish hobbyist group to see if anyone is seeking additional stock.

Finally, if your fish is sick, take it to a veterinarian to be euthanized, or speak to a vet about humane options for home euthanization.

---

5 "Invasive Lionfish Drive Atlantic Coral Reef Fish Declines," John L. Akins, Aleksandra Maljkovi?, and Isabelle M. Càté, Plos One, accessed January 2016. journals.plos.org/plosone/article?id=10.1371/journal. pone.0032596

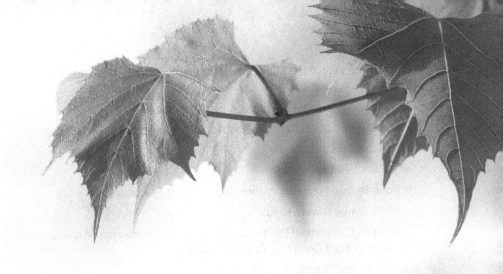

Permissions

Information was graciously provided by the following people and businesses, and was used with their permission:

Abi Cushman, Founder of MyHouseRabbit.com and Brown Bear Creative

Adam Coladipietro and Hilary Barchash, Black Sheep Organics Inc. and Spa Dog Organic Dog Spa

Dr. Adrian Walton, Dewdney Animal Hospital

Alicia Sokolowski, President of AspenClean

Dr. Anthony Pilny, The Center for Avian and Exotic Medicine

Brandy Street, BC SPCA

Brian Feldbloom, Naturally Urban Pet Food Delivery

Dr. Bruce G. Kornreich, Associate Director of Cornell Feline Health Center

Dr. Byron J.S. De la Navarre, Animal House of Chicago, and past President of the Association of Reptilian and Amphibian Veterinarians

Carrie Kish, Director of Reptelligence

Dr. Cathy Lund, City Kitty Veterinary Care for Cats and American Association of Feline Practitioners

Dr. Charlotte Flint, Safety Call International and Senior Consulting Vet for the Pet Poison Helpline

Claire Martin, Climate Critic, Green Party of Canada

Crystal Brisson, Absolutely Clean Personalized Housekeeping Services

Elena Kern, President of the United Mouse Club

Gene Baur, Farm Sanctuary

Dr. Ilona Rodan, American Association of Feline Practitioners

James A. Krause, Rivers to Reef

Jan Jarman, Commercial Feed Consultant and Representative, Association of American Feed Control Officials (AAFCO)

Jennifer Nosek, Modern Dog Magazine

Jesse De Luca, National Reptile Specialist, Rolf C. Hagen Inc.

Dr. Jill Elliot, NY Holistic Vet

Kathy Powelson, Founder and Executive Director of Paws for Hope Animal Foundation

KC Theisen, Director of Pet Care Issues, The Humane Society of the United States (HSUS)

Kimberly Chronister, Vice President, American Mini Pig Association

Lindsay Coulter, Queen of Green, David Suzuki Foundation

Lisa Hutcheon, Co-founder of the Small Animal Rescue Society of BC

Marcella Paraskevas-Ramirez, Holistic Animal Practitioner and Educator

Dr. Marty Becker, "America's Veterinarian" and resident vet on the Dr. Oz Show

Dr. Micah Kohles, Oxbow Animal Health's Director of Veterinary Science and Outreach and President of the Association of Exotic Mammal Veterinarians

Mikkel Becker of Mikkel Becker Animal Training

Nancy L. Shepherd, Pig O' My Heart Potbellies and author of Potbellied Pig Parenting

Dr. Nicky Joosting, Vancouver Feline Veterinary Housecall Service

Dr. Peter G. Fisher, owner of Pet Care Veterinary Hospital

Sabine Contreras, Canine Nutrition Consultant, Better Dog Care and The Dog Food Project

Sharon Lea Slack, City Farmer

Sherri Franklin, Founder and Executive Director of Muttville

Susan Thixton, TruthaboutPetFood.com

Dr. Tina Wismer, Medical Director of the American Society for the Prevention of Cruelty to Animals (ASPCA)

Trupanion

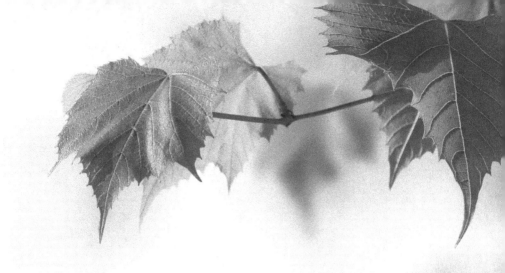

Download Kit

Please enter the URL you see in the box below into your computer web browser to access and download the kit.

www.self-counsel.com/updates/greenpet/16kit.htm

The download kit includes:

- DIY recipes for flee collar, dog shampoo, and more.
- DIY natural cleaning products.
- Build your own dog-waste composter.
- — And more!

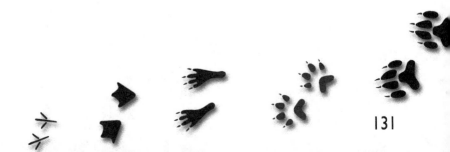